Arthur J. Katz
Abraham Lurie
Carlos Vidal
Editors

Critical Social Welfare Issues
Tools for Social Work and Health Care Professionals

*Pre-publication
REVIEWS,
COMMENTARIES,
EVALUATIONS . . .*

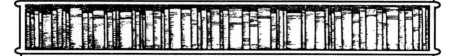

"**A** lively collection on the big social welfare issues by several of social work's big writers and thinkers. It pulls no punches on some of the controversies and totems of the day—'welfare reform,' mental health diagnosis through the DSM-IV, discrimination and prejudice, and the ongoing and growing problem of poverty. A must-read for anyone who wants to understand the real nature of social policy in almost-twenty-first-century America."

Leon Ginsberg, MSW, PhD
Carolina Distinguished Professor,
College of Social Work,
University of South Carolina,
Columbia, SC

"**T**his is a vitally important book not only for social work, social welfare, and health care professionals but also for anyone interested in how civilized and humane societies cope with and treat their poor citizens. The essays in this book have been authored by respected intellectuals and pioneers in the human services field [who] provide a clear and comprehensive examination of the sharply disputed social issues in contemporary America. In that regard they offer thoughtful and timely responses to the recurrent conservative challenge to the concept that government has a responsibility for protection of human life and for maintenance of an adequate level of life quality for all its people.

An excellent introduction to possibilities for re-engineering social work, this is a historically rich and theoretically informed account of the status of social policy, with two common themes running through the specific essays: (1) there has been an extremely conservative shift in social policy toward diminished support for almost every type of entitlement and social program, at both the federal and state levels, which will affect not only minorities, but also immigrants and poor Americans; and (2) this shift dictates that the ways in which social work and social welfare professionals deliver services must now also undergo some changes. The success of this book is due in large measure to the able editorship and authorship of Carlos Vidal and his fellow editors, Arthur Katz and Abe Lurie."

Marcia Bayne Smith, DSW
Assistant Professor,
Urban Studies Department,
Queens College-City University
of New York

More pre-publication
REVIEWS, COMMENTARIES, EVALUATIONS . . .

"The editors have justly entitled their volume *Critical Social Welfare Issues* as their selection of chapters covers a large range of crucial policy, political, value, and systems changes that are impacting on the nature and breadth of social welfare in the United States.

Together this collection provides a useful and important perspective for social work students and practitioners as they seek to understand the evolving context in which services are delivered. It is no longer business as usual. The articles, individually and collectively, serve to promote discussion, generate debate, and encourage the identification of effective responses on the part of the social welfare community based on a beginning series of recommendations offered for professional activism and intervention.

The chapters cover a wide range of substantive, ethical, and professional issues, including HIV testing of newborns; homelessness; the crisis in child welfare; de-professionalization; privatization; managed care; legal regulation and accreditation; and cultural diversity. The result is a panoramic view of the causes and consequences of change in the social welfare system.

In sum, this collection serves to challenge our thinking about critical issues and their solutions and to reinforce social work's mandate to mobilize for action within the context of political and economic realities. To be effective in this endeavor, social workers must be willing to call into question our professional beliefs and bias and recognize that old ways of doing business must be recast within the driving forces of today's world. This book makes a significant contribution to defining the essence of the forces that define and will further redefine American social welfare."

Margaret Gibelman, DSW
Professor and Director,
Doctoral Program,
Wurzweiler School of Social Work,
Yeshiva University,
New York, NY

The Haworth Press, Inc.

Critical Social Welfare Issues
Tools for Social Work and Health Care Professionals

HAWORTH Social Work Practice
Carlton E. Munson, DSW, Senior Editor

Critical Social Welfare Issues
Tools for Social Work and Health Care Professionals

Arthur J. Katz
Abraham Lurie
Carlos Vidal
Editors

The Haworth Press
New York • London

The Haworth Press, Inc., 10 Alice Street, Binghamton, NY 13904-1580

Cover design by Marylouise E. Doyle.

Library of Congress Cataloging-in-Publication Data

Critical social welfare issues : tools for social work and health care professionals / Arthur J. Katz, Abraham Lurie, Carlos Vidal, editors.
     p. cm.
    Includes bibliographical references and index.
    ISBN 0-7890-0161-6 (alk. paper)
    1. Public welfare–Government policy–United States. 2. Social service–Government policy–United States. 3. Child welfare–United States. 4. Medical care–United States. 5. Medical policy–United States. 6. United States–Social policy. 7. United States–Economic policy. I. Katz, Arthur J. II. Lurie, Abraham. III. Vidal, Carlos (Carlos M.)
HV91.C77 1997
361.973–dc21

                                                97-9241
                                                  CIP

CONTENTS

ABOUT THE EDITORS

Arthur J. Katz, PhD, is Professor at the School of Social Welfare in the Health Sciences Center of the State University of New York at Stony Brook. He has taught and held leadership positions at several other universities, including Adelphi University, the Jewish Theological Seminary of America, and the University of Kansas. Dr. Katz has held numerous positions for the NASW, including National President, Vice President of the New York City Chapter, Member of the National Board of Directors, and Chair of the National Political Action Committee. He has also served as Executive Director of the Council on Social Work Education in Washington, DC, and as U.S. Representative to the Permanent Council of the International Federation of Social Workers. He has been a research, educational, or program consultant to several organizations in New York.

Abraham Lurie, PhD, is Professor at the School of Social Welfare in the Health Sciences Center of the State University of New York at Stony Brook and Professor Emeritus at Adelphi University. Dr. Lurie is a Diplomate Clinical Social Work (NASW) and Training Coordinator of Mental Health. He also serves as a consultant to the Mental Health Association in Mineola, New York, and as Board Director and First Board President for Variety Pre-Schoolers in Syosset, New York. He has served as a consultant, board member, or director for several other organizations in New York.

Carlos M. Vidal, PhD, is Clinical Associate Professor and Assistant Dean for the Offices of Field Instruction and Student Services/Admissions at the School of Social Welfare in the Health Sciences Center of the State University of New York at Stony Brook. A longtime activist and leader in the interest of the Hispanic/Latino community, Dr. Vidal researches and lectures extensively on the issues of program planning and research and development. His devotion to community service to the Town of Islip and Suffolk County (New York) has been recognized by numerous awards. In

1994, Dr. Vidal received the New York State Governor's Citation for Hispanic Americans of Distinction. He has served on the Minority Commission of the Council on Social Work Education and as the first Chairperson of the Suffolk County Hispanic Advisory Board. Dr. Vidal has published several articles and reports on Hispanic/Latino issues.

Contributors

Mimi Abramovitz, DSW, Professor of Social Work, Hunter College School of Social Work

Andrew Billingsley, Professor and Chair, Department of Family Studies, University of Maryland, College Park

Judith S. Bloch, ACSW, Executive Director/Founder, Variety Pre-Schoolers Workshops

Richard A. Cloward, Professor, Columbia University School of Social Work

David Fanshel, DSW, Professor Emeritus, Columbia University School of Social Work

Nilsa S. Gutierrez, MD, Former Director, AIDS Institute, New York State Department of Health

Ann Hartman, Professor Emeritus, Smith College

Kim Hopper, MD, Research Scientist, President, Coalition for the Homeless, Nathan Kline Institute

Lorna S. McBarnette, PhD, Dean, School of Health Technology and Management, State University of New York at Stony Brook

Frances Fox Piven, Professor, City University of New York

Juan Ramos, Associate Director for Prevention, National Institute of Mental Health

Gary Rosenberg, PhD, Senior Vice President, The Mount Sinai Medical Center

Carlos Vidal, PhD, Clinical Associate Professor, School of Social Welfare, State University of New York at Stony Brook

Joseph L. Vigilante, PhD, University Professor of Social Policy, Adelphi University

Acknowledgments

The editors are solely responsible for the selection and editing of the articles in this book. But as most know, a work of this kind is the product of many.

Frances L. Brisbane, Dean of the School of Social Welfare at the State University of New York at Stony Brook, inspired us to develop the course, "Distinguished Lectures in Social Welfare." Her sustained interest and support in the preparation of this work encouraged us and helped to make it possible.

The course was offered to social work students in the School of Social Welfare during the Fall and Winter Semester of 1994–1995, and all students, undergraduate and graduate, on the main campus as well as the Health Science Center were invited to participate. Residents in nearby areas were encouraged through local media to attend as well.

We owe many thanks for the invaluable assistance of Florence Graziano, Administrative Assistant, and Sally Brown, Secretary, who despite their heavy job responsibilities took on the extra chores of the administrative work involved in the preparation of this manuscript.

And finally, we are grateful to the authors of the articles who agreed to have their lectures edited and published in this book.

Foreword

It is with great pride and pleasure that we are publishing *Critical Social Welfare Issues: Tools for Social Work and Health Care Professionals,* edited by Arthur Katz, Abraham Lurie, and Carlos Vidal, as part of our Haworth Social Work Textbook Program titled *Practice in Action.* This book genuinely fits the category of practice in action. The collection of articles by leading national and international authorities in the social work profession makes a substantial and lasting contribution to our social work practice knowledge. The authors who have contributed to this volume are some of the most experienced practitioners in the profession, and their insights and observations can serve as guideposts for all who work in the broad areas of practice covered in this book. We hope you find the book enlightening and stimulating.

Carlton E. Munson, PhD

Introduction

In the Fall of 1994, the School of Social Welfare of the State University of New York at Stony Brook instituted a Distinguished Lecturers Series in an effort to enrich the regular ongoing curriculum offerings of the BSW (bachelor of social work) and MSW (masters of social work) programs. The goal of this series was to bring to the campus nationally recognized and outstanding social work and allied health care scholars and practitioners to meet with students and faculty and to present and discuss with them current critical issues in social welfare and social work. The papers that resulted from this effort, delivered by the lecturers, represent the content of this volume.

The results of election day 1994 brought a sense of consternation and crisis to the ranks of social workers and other health care professionals closely identified with social welfare. Given the unexpected triumph of the conservative wing of the Republican party culminating in control of both federal legislative houses as well as state governorships and legislatures, the immediate expectation was that there would be a massive frontal attack on the American social welfare system. Those concerned were not disappointed. The conservative think tanks had been preparing for this opportunity for several decades during the period of Democratic-controlled Congresses. Plans for legislation that were already in the files were dusted off and put into the hopper. However, these were not to be merely adjustments and/or redesigning of programs but rather radical reformulations of the role of government's responsibility and concern for the well-being of those in need. Particularly targeted was the role of the federal government in this area with reference to eliminating the commitment to the federal entitlement concept. As this lecture series unfolded, the crisis in the American social welfare institution deepened and worsened. The requests for waivers from the states to demonstrate "new and innovative" approaches to containing and cutting the costs of income-maintenance programs multiplied in numbers, and the methods to severely limit benefits and eligibility became more bold. The approaches were neither new nor innovative, but rather represented an historically regressive attempt to drastically reduce public expenditures in order to make good the election promises of Republicans to slash taxes for the upper-income constituencies. Under the rubric of ending dependency and eliminating waste and fraud, the most concentrated and severe attack upon the federal welfare system was instituted as part of the "Contract with America." In many states, a rush of waivers were requested to allow for imposition of time limits for recipients, freezing benefits regardless of additional children, elimination of general assistance, workfare without adequate child care or medical benefits, and eliminating benefits for noncitizens among others.

The drastic budget cuts advanced for all of the domestic social programs would provide for the slow strangulation of such benefits and services in the event that the large-scale move to block grant the funding to the states through other legislation progressed too slowly. By this time, the attempt to reformulate the health system of the nation in terms of a national policy was already a failed endeavor. It was clear that comprehensive health-care financing restructuring to guarantee universal coverage fell victim once again to the combined forces of the for-profit health insurance industry, corporate power, and the organized medical profession.

Within this context the lecturers responded to the call to identify critical issues for social welfare and the profession of social work. On a number of vital fronts, it was indeed then and still is now a time of crisis for the institution of social welfare in the United States and for the American social work profession.

In presenting a political-economy analysis of the current welfare-bashing environment, Cloward and Piven conclude that the mainstream analysts ". . . began to recognize that income-maintenance programs had weakened capital's ability to depress wages by the traditional means of intensifying economic insecurity. . . . In effect, social programs altered the terms of struggle between capital and labor." Slashing income-support programs is an effort, therefore, to restore labor discipline.

As of this writing (1996), the welfare reform law enacted by Congress and signed by the President has demonstrated the prescient comments by Cloward and Piven. The results of the law tend to support their thesis that there is indeed a class war—a war against the poor.

Kim Hopper, in examining the crisis in homelessness, discusses a number of significant issues utilizing a radical view. Shelter and housing, Hopper maintains, have never solved homelessness: ". . . to speak simply of 'affordability' begs the question of livelihood: What are people to do after they awake in the morning having moved from being privileged homeless to merely poor?" Hopper invokes the "abeyance process" in his analysis. He laments the disappearance of "virtual work" for redundant people who might otherwise have posed a disruptive threat to the social order. The domains of housing and labor are linked, and Hopper questions how homelessness should in the future be classified as a social problem.

In looking at the crisis in American child welfare, David Fanshel concludes from his own research that the all-time high poverty rate of 26 percent for children under age six "is having devastating consequences on young children and adolescents . . . those seeking draconian changes in the provision of income maintenance to the poor rarely talk about what will happen to the children whose mothers are targeted for the harsh penalties . . . ."

Turning to the arena of health and the crisis of HIV, Nilsa Gutierrez takes a stand on one of the most controversial health policy questions, namely, the HIV testing of newborns. Discussing both sides of the issue, she makes a strong case for opposition to mandatory testing and is convinced that "the best care for children will come from voluntary prenatal counseling and testing of mothers." Unfortunately, the relevance of her comments can be gauged by the enactment of recent legislation in New York State which provides for a comprehensive testing program for HIV (human immuno deficiency virus) and HIV antibodies for all infants born in New York State.

In Andrew Billingsley's thoughtful and well-documented presentation on the changing structure of African-American families, he is critical of the generalizations about the family patterns that often degenerate into stereotypes. The great diversity in African-American families, he maintains, can never be appreciated if public concentration is placed on the low-income unemployed alone, or on single-parent families alone. "In an often myopic focus on the family as an institution, they (analysts) ignore its interdependence with the institutional structure of the black community and with the systems of the larger society."

Mimi Abramovitz focuses on the current attempts to place women at the heart of blame for the problems of the underclass. She maintains that conservative theorists of poverty who are currently influential in the welfare reform debate in policy arenas focus blame for American's social and economic problems on women rather than on the profit-motivated enterprise system. The unrelenting attack against AFDC, Abramovitz insists is a mean-spirited attempt to use government funds to regulate the lives of poor women. The AFDC recipient is portrayed as counter to mainstream cultural values, preferring dependency to work, cheating the government, having children for the extra money, encouraging out-of-wedlock births, causing family breakdown, and generally participating in irresponsible behavior.

She ends with a challenge to the social work profession, which in large part she suggests "has been seduced or co-opted by behavioral explanations of social problems." The use of terms such as "underclass," "welfare dependency," and "culture of poverty," which have become part of professional language, Abramovitz maintains, has made social workers "hostages to the negative metaphors about women, race, and poverty, which these words convey." She offers several viable recommendations for professional activism in her conclusion.

Joseph Vigilante considers the critical issue of the expanding privatization and for-profit thrust in American social welfare and identifies this as a move to an *efficiency* orientation from a *value* orientation. He suggests that the *for-profit* emergency in social welfare represents a reversal of the humanitarian tradition. He states that "massive privatization of human services promises to preserve or worsen the current or unequal accessibility as well as to weaken a long-established commitment to the basic morals and values of a free society." The guarantee of universal institutionalized human services, Vigilante maintains, is not possible in a market economy but must be seen as the "business of government." In his philosophical and historical analysis of this issue, he identifies and discusses four value-critical assumptions that require attention. A key suggestion is to abandon the efficiency orientation in social policy for a value orientation. Vigilante also recommends a paradigm shift in social work from the *scientific* to the *heuristic*.

Juan Ramos sees the critical issues for the social work profession as being lodged in the areas of legal regulation and accreditation. These are identified as "obstacles to service delivery." He raises the following question: "How can the infrastructure of the profession [of social work] be sensitized to the need for self-analysis and change?" Ramos also identifies a crisis in the profession's reluctance, "to seriously engage in effective research to validate its body of knowledge and to create new knowledge." Such reluctance, he maintains, leads to the questioning of social work's competence among policymakers as well as consumers. He asserts that a great opportunity for the profession to redefine itself was missed as the nation moved out of the cold war ethos with the dissolution of the Soviet Union. Social work still continues to be seen as a liberal and even radical profession with "leftist" leanings by policymakers. Such leanings are somehow equated with "socialistic" thinking.

Public health is the area in which the social work profession needs to concentrate in the near future, he suggests, but credibility is an issue here as well. Ramos asserts that a number of social problems have been "medicalized" since resources are more easily garnered under that rubric. He argues that social work has much to contribute to service delivery in such areas as homelessness, HIV management, and violence. Questions need to be raised about managed care and privatization of health care services that have no commitment to cultural sensitivity and operate without cultural competence.

Ramos attempts a critical analysis of legal regulation and the accreditation systems of both social agencies and social work education in relation to concern for the value of diversity. He questions whether or not the current policies driving legal regulation and accreditation "match the needs of the people who are to be served by these policies." He suggests that accreditation standards for all human service programs and for social work education should require a significant amount of cultural-diversity content and that state examinations for licensing and certification also contain such a series of content questions.

Ramos concludes with an appeal for a greater research commitment by the profession. He claims, "There seems to be within the profession an antiscience, anti-intellectual and antiresearch sentiment. Effective mental health intervention needs more than an art form; it needs a scientific base."

Gary Rosenberg defines the most critical issue in the current health care scene as managed care, and he believes there are major implications for social work practice in the health system. He traces the evolution of financing in the health care system and sees the direct contracting between insurers and providers, including capitation payments, as a continuing phenomenon that includes risk taking by physicians and hospitals as the for-profit dynamic becomes stronger.

A dilemma for the social work profession is already surfacing as the future scenario emerges. Hospitals, where most social workers are currently employed, will no longer offer the same employment opportunities. Rosenberg projects that the future focus of action for health care will not be the hospital but rather the community settings, i.e., the primary care offices, the ambulatory care facilities, and satellite community health centers. Rosenberg gives an historical review of health care system development in this nation and discusses the limitations of managed care in the current evolutionary development. He points out the mechanisms by which managed-care companies contain costs and maximize profits. These mechanisms also function to limit access to services and often lessen quality of service. He states, "It is very difficult to track professional accountability in this arena of managed care." As for the future status of social work practice in the health arena, Rosenberg sees practice moving into continuous care systems with patients becoming more active participants in treatment, "The move will force social workers to deal with populations since managed care deals with people on that level." He recommends that social work education include content on social epidemiology and health status as well as other topics such as community health care.

The most promising future domains for social work in the health industry are work with the chronically ill in the community and the aging population with the goals of preventing disability and improving the quality of life. He maintains that in every community social workers can contribute to enhancing the programs for improving community health.

Given cost-containment and profit-maximizing imperatives there is a grave question of whether or not the managed-care system will support such efforts.

Lorna McBarnette also addresses the new developments in health care and its potential effects upon the traditional professions and disciplines that provide services. She points out that in the national debate on reforming the health care system, cost containment and efficiency have taken priority over access and quality. As a result, health professionals have become targets and find themselves in adversarial positions with hospitals, health insurance companies, and managed-care companies. Given the preference for routinization and rationalization of professional activity as a way of managing and controlling their work, there is a sense of "deprofessionalization" emerging.

McBarnette suggests that social work is currently in a very vulnerable position. Social work's knowledge base is of an "abstract nature" enabling it to avoid external quality assessment. This may prompt external intervention based on the lack of certification that the knowledge base has utility. She maintains that major purchasers of health care will look for cheaper "substitutes" in all of the disciplines and that social work will need strong advocacy support from its national organization to avoid this inexorable push for deprofessionalization by the managed-care system. Since other professions see a similar threat, they may seek to enhance their positions by competing with social work for certain functions. Consumer self-help groups and the so-called "indigenous" workers are also competitive substitutes.

McBarnette calls for a "well-planned effort to delineate the scope of practice and create professional boundaries." In the area of mental health where psychiatry, psychology, and social work psychotherapy often overlap, she identifies an historical problem. However, in reference to managed care and cost containment, it would seem that social work psychotherapy, being the cheapest provider, would have less to fear. Yet, with a lack of verified utility of social work psychotherapy practice, could other less expensive substitutes not be discovered? A discussion of the changing health care environment and the organization of the medical care sector leads McBarnette to the conclusion that "a plethora of differing concerns" among professional groups exists and that professional groups exercise power to enforce their monopoly and escape external controls. Occupational licensing is the most visible way of establishing an occupational monopoly, and she strongly supports the licensing effort for social work, which would protect not only the title—as in certification—but the scope of practice as well.

A series of strategies is suggested. Particular reference is made to creating a context for societal revaluing of the profession: "If the public has difficulty comprehending what social workers do or the curriculum by which they are trained, it is understandable that they will not value it." McBarnette calls for a united front by all health care professions to counter the negative effects of privatization and managed care in their drive to maximize profits at the expense of access to and quality of care.

Judith Bloch leads us into a discussion of secondary prevention in mental health. Special education at the preschool level, Bloch proposes, can have significant positive effects on the future development of troubled children. She documents an ever-increasing population of disturbed preschoolers who are likely to become violent juveniles. They have multiple risk factors and are often neglected, abused, and neurologically impaired. Many are the products of a series of unsuccessful foster-care placements. "Mother blaming" seems to dominate the dialogue in both professional and public arenas. Bloch points out some promising interventions in two federally funded programs, Special Education for Preschoolers and Head Start. Both interventions have reported significant positive outcomes, the key to which has been home-school collaboration. This model puts into practice proposals that child development is advanced by frequent interactions with professional providers, goal consensus between settings, and supportive linkages.

Preschool special education became a mandated entitlement in 1986 but is currently, like most others, under heavy siege as the search for budget-slashing items is underway. The concept of entitlement seems currently to be an anathema of the current majority of federal policymakers, including many Democrats.

The vast overhaul of federal welfare policy includes severe limitations on immigrants and the children of immigrants, many of whom are Hispanic. As Vidal indicates, the Hispanic population in the United States has increased almost seven times as fast as the rest of the population. This population is a diverse group whose struggle for economic and social survival has now been made even more difficult. They will require the utmost sensitivity from those who are involved in helping them gain self-sufficiency and empowerment. To do this, health care professionals, in particular, need to understand the characteristics of Hispanic culture, including Hispanics' sense of oppression by a dominant culture and their fierce commitment to their children and their family systems.

The chapter also reflects the complexities of working with the challenge of diversity within the Hispanic community, mirroring similar issues of the many cultural entities within our current national population.

Ann Hartman argues that social workers historically have been concerned with the issue of power and how it affects human relationships. The strong commitment to self-determination is one example. As social workers came to realize that self-determination in a highly competitive market society was often an empty phrase without access to power, the concept of empowerment for clients became a goal. Yet client empowerment presupposes the professional's readiness to relinquish power. Hartman discusses the sources of power that often overlap and reinforce each other. The one source that she suggests is cherished by all professions is expertise and knowledge: "The power of expertise exists at the heart of our professional practice, but it is the power source with which social workers tend to be the least aware . . . ."

Hartman discusses social constructivism and postmodernism and their challenge to social work's use of expertise power and its long-held truisms. There are multiple truths as there are multiple observers. She refers to Foucalt's concept of power/knowledge "where those in power define the truth and in turn, the truth is supported by those in power." An example in social work knowledge-building is the disappearance from the literature of detailed case examples. The "N's of one," which represented lived experiences in these case examples, were not considered "scientific knowledge." She views the *Diagnostic and Statistical Manual of Mental Disorders* (DSM) as part of "global unitary knowledge," which turns out to be not only descriptive but prescriptive. Other examples in social work practice of the power/knowledge imperative is the dramatic incest story and the definition of homosexuality as a disease in the old DSM as well as the adoption story. The "insurrection of subjugated knowledge" (Foucalt) provides a way for a reappraisal of mainstream thinking about social problems.

Hartman makes a number of provocative recommendations for social work practitioners and social work education, all of which deserve significant consideration. They may be considered controversial and in some cases at odds with the thoughts of other contributors to this volume. To follow her lead, should social workers give up the expert role in favor of the "not knowing" position? Should students be taught to be "informed rather than knowing" listeners? Should we learn to deconstruct theories by looking at their context?

Hartman's final conclusions are substantive, insightful, and in the philosophical vanguard for the emerging paradigm of future social work practice, one which can fully recognize and advance the seminal value underpinnings of this profession in the context of current societal dynamics.

Each day, the media brings increasing evidence that many of the issues discussed in these chapters are vibrant, timely, and of professional significance to providers and to insurers. Health care providers such as hospital systems, physicians, and insurance companies are merging into huge conglomerates challenging the largest industrial giants in terms of capitalization and assets. Recently, the projected health care complex of the Mt. Sinai Hospital and New York University Center in New York City plus the North Shore Hospital Network in Long Island may well become the largest medical center in the United States with the largest number of hospital beds.

It is clear that the American institution of social welfare and the profession of social work—its chief representative discipline—as well as other health care professions are once again under severe philosophical and political attack. Such crises are not historically new, and each time they occur, there are ominous warnings about the imminent dangers of institutional collapse. The threat currently seems to be coming not only from governmental forces focused on tax reductions and right-wing ideologies, but for the first time from the nongovernment sector, the for-profit market system, which is projecting huge profits from health care, education, and corrections among other social welfare arenas that were formerly not targeted from market entrepreneurial enterprises.

Is this the factor that makes the current crisis a more formidable one? After all, there have been similar pronouncements of social welfare and social work demise occurring each time a conservative Republican power force came into being either at the White House level (Nixon and Reagan) or at the congressional level (Gingrich and others). This nation's social welfare system is a major industry commanding a huge slice of the American pie. As the services sector of the U.S. economy constantly expands and its percentage of the gross domestic product increases, it is being targeted for takeover. The target, however, this time is not another corporation but the federal government first and state governments later, once block-granting is completed.

The phenomenon is not a new one, of course, having had its major impetus during the Johnson administration with purchase of service contracting with "for-profit" organizations given entry into the human services system. Another target is the private, nonprofit sector, beginning with hospitals among other health and human service areas. Health care professionals, including social workers, with entrepreneurial aspirations are participating actively. Witness the increasing number of social workers entering or preparing for private practice in solo or corporate human services enterprises as partners and/or investors. There is ongoing informal discussion among professional social workers on the question, "Is the market system the wave of the future and the way to go?"

To Abramovitz's concern about social workers buying into such professional antithetical code words of the dominant discourse such as "welfare dependency," "Culture of Poverty," and "underclass" can be added "cost containment," "market efficiency," and "government intrusion."

The fundamental premise upon which the modern American social welfare system has been built and with which it has most successfully functioned is that of institutionalized governmental responsibility at the highest level for the well-being of its citizens. Simply put, it is federal entitlements for protection of human life and an adequate quality-of-life maintenance. It is the hallmark of every contemporary society that claims the virtue of civilization and humanity.

Arthur Katz
Abraham Lurie

Chapter 1

Class War and Welfare Reform

Richard A. Cloward
Frances Fox Piven

The program we call welfare provides a bare subsistence income to more than four million women raising children. It costs $22 billion dollars, less than 1 percent of the federal budget, and only 2 or 3 percent of most state budgets. Yet this small program has become the target of big guns, both intellectual guns and political ones. Liberals and conservatives agree that welfare is the nation's major problem, is bad for the country, and is bad for the poor. Presumably, it drains public budgets and reduces work effort. And by allowing poor mothers to opt out of paid work, it saps their initiative, and nourishes cultural and psychological disabilities. As a result, welfare is said to worsen poverty, not to speak of its ostensible role in fostering crime, illegitimacy, and the growth of an "underclass." The proposed remedies vary, but they usually involve cutting benefits and forcing mothers into the labor market.

These themes have been developed in an enlarging stream of conservative literature: Nathan Glazer's "The Limits of Social Policy" (1971) and Martin Anderson's *Welfare: The Political Economy of Welfare Reform in the United States* (1978) were among the opening salvos. George Gilder's *Wealth and Poverty* (1981), Ken Auletta's *The Underclass* (1982), and Charles Murray's *Losing Ground* (1984) expanded the attack. 1992 was a banner year for the conservative assault on welfare, with the publication of Lawrence M. Mead's *The New Politics of Poverty: The Nonworking Poor in America*, Daniel Patrick Moynihan's "How the Great Society 'Destroyed the American Family,'" by which he means the black family, and Micky Kaus's *The End of Equality*. As for liberals, they rallied around David Elwood's *Poor Support* (1988), which differed from conservative proposals mainly in that it placed greater emphasis on education and training before expelling mothers from the rolls.

To cope with these new issues, critics of welfare urge putting women to work. Their claims for this reform are as unreal as their depiction of the problem. Near miraculous social and cultural transformations are predicted once welfare mothers join the labor market. Cohesion will be restored to family and community, crime and other aberrant behaviors will disappear, and poverty will decline. Mickey Kaus (1992), who advocates replacing welfare with a WPA-type job program, invokes a grand historical parallel: "Underclass culture can't survive the end of welfare any more than feudal culture could survive the advent of capitalism" (p. 129).

Not unexpectedly, the 1992 presidential campaign featured welfare reform. Clinton promised to "end welfare as we know it." Polls showed that this was Clinton's most popular campaign issue. There have since been various studies and commissions, and the recommendations are all similar: provide some training, develop more workfare programs coupled with new sanctions, and impose a two-year lifetime limit on welfare.

WORK AND THE NEW CLASS WAR

There is no economically and politically practical way to replace welfare with work, given the contemporary conditions of the contemporary labor market. After the great post–World War II boom, which lasted until the early 1970s, the American economy went into decline. For a quarter of a century after World War II, the American economy enjoyed unparalleled expansion, and economists wrote books with titles such as *The Affluent Society* (Galbraith, 1958). But wages peaked in 1973, and then declined, a response in part to intensified competition from Europe and Japan, and later from newly industrializing countries, which devastated the auto, steel, textiles, electronics, and machine tool industries in the United States, reducing manufacturing employment from 30 percent of the workforce in 1960 to less than 20 percent in 1990. Meanwhile, the service sector grew, with its low wages and meager benefits, and economists wrote books with titles such as *The Deindustrialization of America* (Bluestone and Harrison, 1982), or *A Future of Lousy Jobs: The Changing Structure of U.S. Wages* (Burtless, 1990), or *The Age of Diminished Expectations: U.S. Economy Policy in the 1990s* (Krugman 1990).

In response to these global changes, which threatened profitability, American business declared "class war." Businesses pillaged the economy. They shored up profits by closing plants and moving capital out of the old high-wage industrial regions and into low-wage regions here and abroad. They turned to speculation—in real estate and in the financial markets, including mergers and leveraged buyouts of industrial assets. They looted the multibillion-dollar defense-contracting sector and the savings and loan industry. Following Reagan's election in 1980, business taxes were cut, depriving the Federal Treasury of two trillion dollars by 1992 (Sasser, 1993).

Most important, business abandoned its postwar policy of accommodation with labor, using the threat of plant closings accompanied by capital flight to strike fear in the hearts of workers. Capital's power over labor was enlarged all the more by other changes. One was the end of the Cold War, and the gradual shrinking of defense employment. Another was the laying off of workers by corporations seeking to reduce costs. And still another was the flooding of the labor market by great numbers of women who were trying to shore up family income, as well as by millions of immigrants from Asia, Mexico, and other Latin American countries. Unemployment averaged 4.4 percent in the 1950s, 4.7 percent in the 1960s, 6.1 percent in the 1970s, 7.2 percent in the 1980s, and job prospects look little better so far in the 1990s. Consequently, every measure of labor's power fell. Overall, the percentage of unionized workers in the private sector fell from 29.1 percent in 1970 to 12 percent in 1990 (Brody, 1992, p. 33).

With labor cowed, business could make enormous cuts in its permanent workforce, hire temporary and part-time workers instead, and slash wages and benefits. By the 1990s, 30 million people—over a quarter of the U.S. labor force—were working in jobs outside the regular full-time workforce. Nonsupervisory personnel (who make up 81 percent of the workforce) suffered an hourly wage decline of 15 percent between 1973 and 1992.[1]

The spoils reaped by business in the war against labor were large enough to constitute an historic shift in the distribution of income and well-being in American society. Overall, the simultaneous growth of poverty and wealth was unprecedented in the twentieth century (Krugman, 1990, p. 20). This was partly a simple and direct consequence of lowered taxes for the rich and social program cuts for poorer groups.

Between 1977 and 1992, the poorest tenth lost 20.3 percent of its posttax income. The top tenth gained 40.9 percent, the top 5 percent gained 59.7 percent, and the top 1 percent gained 135.7 percent (see Table 1.1).

And poverty increased. By the official measure, poverty had fallen from 22.4 percent in 1959 (39.5 million people) to a low of 11.6 percent in 1977 (24.7 million people). Then it rose to 14.2 per-

TABLE 1.1. Changes in Posttax Family Income, 1977-1992
(in constant 1992 dollars)

Decile Rank	Changes in Income
poorest tenth	− 20.3%
second	− 11.2
third	− 10.9
fourth	− 9.8
fifth	− 10.5
sixth	− 4.7
seventh	− 1.0
eighth	3.8
ninth	8.4
richest tenth	40.9
top 5 percent	59.7
top 1 percent	135.7
all deciles	− 9.1

Source: Congressional Budget Office.

cent in 1991 (35.7 million people), the highest level in a quarter of a century. Moreover, the official poverty measure greatly underestimated poverty. When the poverty line was first calculated in the 1960s, the average family spent one-third of its income on food, and the poverty line was set at three times food costs, adjusted for family size. By 1990, food costs had dropped to one-sixth of the average family budget because other components—such as housing—had inflated at far higher rates. If the 1990 official poverty line of $13,360 for a family of four had been recalculated to reflect changes in the real costs of these components, it would have been about 155 percent of the official rate, or $21,700. By that measure, poverty soared. From the same 22.4 percent in 1959 (39.5 million people), it fell to a low of 17.3 percent in 1972 (35.6 million people), and then rose to 25.6 percent in 1989 (62.8 million people)—or to almost twice the numbers shown by the official indicator.[2]

The most dramatic measure of the reordered class structure was wealth accumulation—aggregate household assets, whether homes and other real estate, stock, bonds, paintings, jewelry, or yachts. Studies by the Federal Reserve show that between 1983 and 1989—the core Reagan years—the richest one percent of families increased their share of net private wealth from 31 to 37 percent, and they did so at the expense of all other social strata. The share of the next richest 9 percent fell from 35 to 31 percent, and the bottom 90 percent lost 1 percent, from 33 to 32 percent.[3] In a characteristically opaque statement, Alan Greenspan, chair of the Federal Reserve, remarked of this finding that material distribution has become "more dispersed"; Claudia Goldin, an economic historian, put the data in perspective when she said the following: "Inequality is at its highest since the great leveling of wages and wealth during the New Deal and World War II."[4] Plainly, business won the war against workers.

WELFARE AND THE NEW CLASS WAR

Even as this degradation of workers worsened, all eyes turned toward welfare, and one heard a growing chorus of antiwelfare rhetoric about the "cycle of dependency." Thus, Daniel Patrick Moynihan grandiosely proclaimed to the press that "just as unemployment was the defining issue of industrialism, dependency is becoming the defining issue of postindustrial society."[5] Lawrence A. Mead (1992) bemoaned the way that "dependency" signals "the end of the Western tradition" (p. 237). The national press announced that "dependency" had reached "epidemic proportions." By these accounts, rising unemployment, declining wage levels, and disappearing fringe benefits need not concern anyone. "The old issues were economic and structural," according to Mead (1992), and "the new ones are social and personal" (p. 221).

What is not understood is that this attack on welfare and, relatedly, on other income programs is an extremely significant part of the new class war. To see the connection, it is useful to remember an old Marxist idea, that the unemployed constitute a "reserve army of labor" used by capitalists to weaken and divide the proletariat. Desperation pits the unemployed against the still-employed, thus weakening labor's bargaining power, but income security programs reduce unemployment and temper desperation. These programs remove millions of people from the labor market and protect millions of others from the ravages of unemployment. The consequence is to tighten labor markets and reduce fear among those still in the market, and thus to strengthen workers in bargaining with employers over wages and working conditions.

Not surprisingly, programs with such potentially large effects generate conflict. They also, from time to time, spur a good deal of highblown and usually unilluminating commentary by the experts of the day. A main theme, in the past as now, is that public income programs do more harm than good by leading to indolence and demoralization among the poor. Reams of such criticism accompanied the passage of the English poor law reform in the 1830s, which eliminated "outdoor" relief in favor of the workhouse. Writing more than a century later, and in a far more compassionate spirit than is typical, Karl Polanyi (1957) nevertheless reiterated the same arguments in his analysis of the 1795 Speenhamland relief-in-aid-of-wages plan, inaugurated by the landed nobility in response to the rising civil disorder among the peasantry who had been displaced from their traditional agricultural occupations during the latter half of the eighteenth century. Under this system, the poor were required to work for whatever wages they could get, with relief authorities supplementing their incomes. Polanyi concluded that this arrangement produced massive destitution and misery because the main effect of the allowance system was to depress wages below the subsistence level. With that conclusion, he left the impression that it was the giving of relief that depressed wages and produced misery.

What Polanyi failed to see was that the debilitating consequences of the Speenhamland relief-in-aid-of-wages system were not the result of income guarantees, but of the use of relief to flood the labor market with surplus workers, thus empowering employers in bargaining over wages. By contrast, a relief system that takes surplus workers out of the labor market empowers those still working in bargaining with employers.

In the current period, business advisors seem to understand this, even if the Left does not. Concern about the impact of public income programs on wages became evident in the 1970s. Policymakers were troubled: Unemployment rose in the late 1960s and early 1970s, but wages did not fall. This contradicted the common wisdom among economists that unemployment and wage levels vary inversely—a relationship embodied not only in the reserve army thesis, but in the neo-classical formula known as the "Phillips Curve" (Phillips, 1958).[6] Post–World War II government macroeconomic policies were designed with this relationship in mind. Fiscal and monetary policies, by expanding or contracting aggregate demand and by raising or lowering the price of money, enabled government to control wage demands by manipulating levels of unemployment.[7]

For two decades following World War II, the unemployment-wages trade-off varied to order. Cyclical increases in unemployment were matched by the expected fall in the rate of wage increases. In the late 1960s, however, wages spiraled upward despite a 6 percent unemployment level. Barry Bosworth (1980), who later headed Carter's Council on Wage and Price Stability, reported that "wage rate increases had actually accelerated slightly despite the high unemployment" (pp. 60-61). The problem persisted in the early 1970s as unemployment rose to the highest levels since the 1930s, but wages still did not fall. Wage levels appeared to be immune to rising unemployment. Something had happened to disrupt the traditional relationship between unemployment and wage levels, between the supply of labor and the power of labor. In another idiom, the reserve army of labor was no longer performing its historic function.

A good number of economic analysts concluded that the expansion of income-maintenance programs in the late 1960s and early 1970s had insulated wages from the effects of rising unemployment. The extension of social security coverage, together with higher benefits, sharply reduced workforce participation among older people. At any one time, three million women were on the AFDC (Aid to Families with Dependent Children) rolls in the early 1970s, and few of them were then required to participate in welfare-supplemented work. The expansion of the disability programs from less than one million recipients in 1960 to more than four million in 1975 also produced a sizeable drop in labor force participation since many of these people were of prime working age.

Unemployment benefits also shrank the numbers looking for work. In the decades since 1935, coverage was extended to more workers, and benefits were liberalized, most importantly by congressional action extending the duration of coverage during periods of high unemployment. In the recession of 1973-1974, when unemployment rose above 10 percent, the basic 26-week period of coverage was extended to 65 weeks (and many workers displaced from jobs by foreign competition also received benefits under the Trade Adjustment Assistance Act). As a result, two out of three of the 12 million unemployed received benefits during the 1973-1974 downturn. Almost all studies concluded that the availability of unemployment benefits increases the length of unemployment spells (Danziger, Haveman, and Plotnick, 1981). The unemployed could "prolong job search . . . refuse to accept work except at higher offered wages or cease active labor market participation" (Danziger, Haveman, and Plotnick, 1981, p. 46) for a period of months, thus tightening the labor market. Looking at the labor-market effects of all of the social programs taken together, the total hours worked by *all* workers were reduced by between 4.8 and 7 percent.[8] No wonder economists concluded that "a change has taken place" in the unemployment/wages trade-off (Fiedler, 1989, p. 117).

In sum, mainstream analysts (and no matter that they couched their conclusions in the idiom of the Phillips Curve rather than of the reserve army) began to recognize that income-maintenance programs had weakened capital's ability to depress wages by the traditional means of intensifying economic insecurity. Unemployment had thus lost some of its terrors, both for the unemployed and for those still working. In effect, social programs altered the terms of the struggle between capital and labor.

What followed, of course, was an effort to restore labor discipline by slashing the income-support programs. This was no easy matter, given the near universal public support for programs such as social security. In the drawn-out contest that ensued, the Reagan administration sometimes backed off or turned to administrative subterfuge to achieve the cuts it wanted. For some programs, such as social security, the result was something of a standoff. Still, other programs, especially those that affect more vulnerable groups, were badly damaged. Unemployment insurance coverage was severely restricted, for example, through a series of little-understood changes in the law, so that only one in three receive benefits. Nearly a-half million people were removed from the disability rolls (although the courts subsequently ruled that many had been removed illegally). In other programs, new and confusing bureaucratic obstacles were introduced to deter utilization. Their significance is suggested by a series of studies of the food stamp program—by the Urban Institute, the Congressional Budget Office, and the General Accounting Office—which found that only one-third to one-half of all eligible persons were receiving food stamp benefits. An Urban Institute study reported that one-third of those eligible for medicaid, a health insurance program specifically for the poor, were not receiving benefits.

Welfare grant levels fell sharply (in lockstep, we add, with the drop in the minimum wage).[9] AFDC grant levels began to fall when protest subsided at the close of the 1960s as state legislatures generally stopped raising AFDC payments, or even adjusting them for inflation. The result was that benefits lost 42 percent of their purchasing power between 1970 and 1990. By 1990, the maximum benefit was less than half the poverty level in a majority of the states, and less than one-third of that level in a quarter of the states; for a family of three, the daily per capita benefit in the median payment state was $4.00 and as the nation entered recession in 1990, the pace of AFDC cuts actually accelerated (see Table 1.2).[10]

TABLE 1.2. Median State Monthly AFDC Benefit
(for a family of four with no other income)

Year 1990 Dollars	Payment	Constant
1970	$221	$739
1975	264	635
1980	350	552
1985	399	483
1990	432	432
1970-1990 % Change	195%	

However, since Food Stamp benefits were made uniform nation-ally and indexed for inflation by Congress beginning in 1972, they maintained their purchasing power, and partly offset AFDC losses. In constant 1990 dollars, average monthly Food Stamp payments per person rose from $43.50 in 1972 to $61.50 in 1990.[11] Combin-ing payments from AFDC and food stamps, the purchasing power of AFDC families was reduced by about 27 percent between 1972 and 1990.

Throughout this contest, however, and continuing today, the main focus of discussion by politicians and policy intellectuals was less on the range of major social programs that were at issue, and more on the welfare program. It is easy to see why. Welfare, with its ancient connotations of pauperism and its contemporary association with blacks, could easily be made to symbolize the error of the very idea of income-support programs. Also, welfare recipients—most of whom are single mothers, many of whom are minorities, and all of whom are desperately poor—could easily be made to symbolize the failures of character of those who drop out of wage work.

Welfare clients have always suffered the insult of extremely low benefit levels and have always been degraded by the overbearing and punitive procedures of welfare agencies. Now, as public furor over welfare builds, meager benefits are cut, and degrading proce-dures multiply, the moral for Americans who are working more and earning less is clear. There is an even worse fate, an even lower status, than hard and unrewarding work.

Because most AFDC mothers are unskilled, they can only command the lowest wages, a problem that is worsening as wages decline. According to the Census Bureau, there were 14.4 million (or 18 percent) of year-round, full-time workers 16 years of age or older who had annual earnings below the poverty level in 1990, up from 10.3 million (14.6 percent) in 1984, and from 6.6 million (12.3 percent) in 1974.[12] (The Bush administration tried to suppress these findings.)[13] There is no reason to think that most AFDC mothers can become "self-sufficient" when growing millions of workers cannot. In a study of the finances of welfare families, Christopher Jencks and Kathryn Edin (1992) find that "single mothers do not turn to welfare because they are pathologically dependent on handouts or unusually reluctant to work—they do so because they cannot get jobs that pay better than welfare" (p. 204).

Research on work programs supports this. Fred Block and John Noakes (1988) conclude that recipients typically cannot find jobs that pay more than welfare. A review of research conducted by the Center on Budget and Policy Priorities (Porter, 1990) shows that work programs—highly publicized stories of individual successes notwithstanding—do not result in more than a handful of recipients achieving "a stable source of employment that provides enough income for a decent standard of living (at least above the poverty line) and job-related benefits that adequately cover medical needs" (p. 5). Still another general review, this time sponsored by the Brookings Institution (Burtless, 1989), reports that none of the programs succeed in raising earnings by welfare mothers more than $2,000. Schwarz and Volgy (1992) conclude that "No matter how much we may wish it otherwise, workfare cannot be an effective solution" because "low-wage employment riddles the economy": one in seven year-round full-time jobs in 1989, or 11 million jobs, paid less than $11,500 for the year, which was roughly $2,000 below the official poverty line for a family of four (pp. 81, 106).

Another reason to be skeptical about welfare-to-work programs is that, although they are promoted as economy measures, they would in fact be very expensive if anyone actually intended to implement them widely. Administrative costs alone would overshadow any savings from successful job placements. To this must be added the much larger costs of government-subsidized child-care, and health care, especially since the private market is offering fewer benefits to newly hired workers. For example, Medoff (1992) estimates that the proportion of new hires who get health benefits dropped from 23 to 15 percent during the last decade. Jencks (1992) estimates that AFDC mothers working at the minimum wage would have to be given free medical care and at least $5,000 worth of resources to supplement their wages, at a cost in excess of $50 billion, a quixotic sum, which he agreed was unlikely to be appropriated by Congress. Kaus (1992) offers a similar dollar estimate for his recommendation for a mandatory jobs program for the poor. The Congress is certainly not unmindful of these costs as indicated by its endless squabbling over whether health- and day-care benefits to working recipients should be funded at all, or for only four months, or nine months, or twelve months, or whatever.

Given these constraints, the results of the existing work program are predictable enough. Studies show that a substantial proportion of former recipients end up reapplying for welfare because they cannot survive on their earnings, even with welfare supplements, and because temporary child-care and medicaid supports run out, or because of periodic crises such as a job layoff or an illness in the family. During the 1992 presidential campaign, Clinton claimed that 17,000 Arkansas residents had been successfully moved off the AFDC and Food Stamps rolls under a state jobs program between 1989 and 1992. The administrator of the program subsequently acknowledged that many people returned to welfare during that period. So the charade goes on, as experts and politicians promise to put an end to welfare "dependency." None of it seems to make pragmatic sense.

Other professed goals of the work programs are equally irrational, if taken at face value, such as the unsubstantiated assertions that work would transform family structure, community life, and the so-called "culture of poverty." Kaus (1992) insists that "Replacing welfare with work can be expected to transform the entire culture of poverty," including family patterns, because "it's doubtful" that working women would "be willing to share their hard-earned paychecks with nonworking men the way they might have been willing to share their welfare checks," so that "the natural incentives toward the formation of two-parent families will reassert themselves"

(p. 129). However, Kaus presents no data to support the view that the source of a woman's income influences marriage rates. In our judgment, marriage rates might indeed increase were jobs with adequate wages and benefits available to men, as well as to women on welfare who choose to work, but that seems entirely unlikely in view of current economic trends.

It is also doubtful that putting poor women to work would improve the care and socialization of children. Kaus (1992) claims that "[i]f a mother has to set her alarm clock, she's likely to teach her children to set their alarm clocks as well" (p. 129), thus trivializing the real activities of most of these women. Many AFDC mothers with younger children get their children up every morning and, because of the danger in the streets, walk them to school, walk them home, and keep them locked up in their apartments until morning. Forcing these overburdened women to work would mean adding the market job to the exhausting job of maintaining a home without funds or services—while being surrounded by dangerous and disorganized neighborhoods.

Work is also advertised as the way to reverse the deterioration of community life. This is hardly a new idea. The minutes of a meeting of academics, intellectuals, and administrators who met in New York City after Nixon's election in 1968 reported a general consensus that the rising welfare rolls accompanied by spreading urban riots and other manifestations of civil disorder proved that "The social fabric . . . is coming to pieces. It isn't just 'strained' and it isn't just 'frayed'; but like a sheet of rotten canvas, it is starting to rip . . . ." (Moynihan, 1973, p. 76). Converting AFDC to a work system was the remedy; work would restore the social fabric.

Removing women from their homes and neighborhoods would more likely shred the social fabric more. Putting mothers to work would deprive the poor community of its most stable element—of the women, for example, who have mounted campaigns to drive drug dealers from their housing projects and neighborhoods. Sally Hernandez-Pinero, the chairwoman of the New York City Housing Authority, commented on the social roles played by the 75,000 women living and raising children alone in the New York City projects. "Anyone with even a nodding acquaintance with these women knows them for what they are, the sanity of the poor community, resourceful survivors of abandonment, slander, and brutality . . . . In many poor communities, they are the only signatures on the social contract, the glue that keeps our communities from spinning out of control."[14]

None of the critics explains convincingly why these women would contribute more to their communities by taking jobs flipping hamburgers. Nor do they explain why it would not be the better part of public policy to shore up income supports (as we noted earlier, the real value of AFDC benefits has fallen by 43 percent since the early 1970s, and by 27 percent if food stamps are counted), and to shore up social supports for women who are struggling to care for children under the jungle-like conditions of urban poverty. Instead, the family and community work performed by these women—like the family and community work of women more generally—is consistently ignored or devalued.

Of course, many welfare mothers do want to work, and they should have the chance to work. They also should have the training and supportive benefits, such as day care and health care, as well as wage income and supplemental welfare payments that would enable their families to survive in the market. Under such conditions, many would take jobs, and coercion would be unnecessary. As a realistic matter, however, such opportunities are not on the reform agenda. It is the charade of work that is on the agenda.

Despite the record of workfare failures, an aura of optimism continues to permeate the literature on welfare reform. Most experts are convinced that most welfare mothers can achieve self-sufficiency through work and that benign consequences for family and community will ensue. The key to eventual success is to find the proper mix of programs targeted to those who can best benefit from them. As theories and policies proliferate—none of them gaining ascendance for long, since none of them succeed in practice—the search goes on and on for new strategies, or mix of strategies, that will produce the desired outcomes. This occurs, Schram (1992) points out, even though the research data that reformers invoke to justify workfare legislation show that there will be few if any effects, leading him to conclude that these initiatives represent "symbols at the expense of substance."

REINFORCING WORK NORMS
AND THE NEW CLASS WAR

However, the charade is in fact the point. Welfare bashing is an easy political strategy. Politicians are rushing to divert voter discontent by focusing on welfare mothers, a majority of whom are black and Hispanic—and easy scapegoats. Moreover, this sort of appeal draws strength from an inherited political culture, from nineteenth-century ideas about the low morals of the poor, and from nineteenth-century schemes to make the poor shape up by disciplining them.

In other words, politicians are pandering to the currents of race hatred and class hatred in American culture. The reasons are obvious. Political leaders have nothing to say about jobs, about widening economic inequality, about pervasive economic insecurity, or about the broad social demoralization these economic conditions bring in their wake. The public is anxious, but political leaders have neither the ideas nor the courage to speak to that anxiety. Instead, they point the finger of blame at poor women. Politicians have discovered that AFDC moms make good scapegoats.

Not only are people encouraged to blame the poor for their own troubles, but the rituals that degrade welfare recipients reaffirm the imperative of work at a time when wages are down, working conditions worse, and jobs less secure. Kaus (1992) wrote that while we cannot promise the poor who work that "they'll be rich, or even comfortably well-off" (and, he might have added, we cannot even promise them a living wage), "we can promise them respect" because they "would have the tangible honor society reserves for workers" (pp. 138-139). The charade of work-enforcement reform should thus be understood as a symbolic crusade directed to the working poor rather than to those on relief, and the moral conveyed is the shame of the dole and the virtue of labor, no matter the job and no matter the pay.

NOTES

1. Data supplied by D. Y. Henwood (Ed.), 1994, *Left Business Review*, New York.
2. Schwarz and Volgy, p. 42, and Table 6, p. 62.

3. Relevant studies of wealth redistribution are summarized in *Dollars and Sense*, October 1992, 32.

4. Both Greenspan and Goldin are quoted in *The New York Times*, April 20, 1991.

5. Moynihan, *The New York Times*, December 9, 1991, p. A13.

6. This formula included prices as well as wages.

7. Unionization and minimum wage laws modify but do not eliminate these effects.

8. See Danziger, Haveman, and Plotnick, 1981, p. 996, for the lower estimate, and Robert Lampman, 1979, for the higher one.

9. Even *The New York Times*, June 8, 1991, p. A15, noted the coincidence, reporting that the 27 percent drop in the real value of welfare and food stamp benefits over the past two decades roughly matches the 23 percent drop in the value of the minimum wage.

10. See press release reports issued by the Center on Budget and Policy Priorities, September 8, 1992, and February 1993.

11. *1992 Green Book, Overview of Entitlement Programs.* (May 15, 1992). Committee on Ways and Means, U.S. House of Representatives. Washington, DC: U.S. Government Printing Office. Table 12, p. 1639.

12. U.S. Census, May 1992.

13. Writing in *Barrons* (May 18, 1992) in the article, "Numbers Game: A Census Bureau Wage Report Takes Five Months to Surface," Maggie Mahar tells the whole story.

14. From an unpublished speech at Columbia University in 1992, with thanks to Val Coleman.

REFERENCES

Anderson, M. (1978). *Welfare: The political economy of welfare reform in the United States*. Stanford, CA: Hoover Institution.

Auletta, K. (1982). *The Underclass*.

Block, F., and J. Noakes. (1988). The politics of new-style workfare. *Socialist Review,* 18.

Bluestone, B., and B. Harrison. (1982). *The Deindustrialization of America*. New York: Basic Books.

Bosworth, B. (1980). Re-establishing an economic consensus: An impossible agenda? *Daedalus*, 109, 3.

Brody, D. (1992). The breakdown of labor's social contract. *Dissent*, Winter.

Burtless, G. (1989). The effect of reform on employment, earnings and income. In P. Cottingham and D. Ellwood (Eds.), *Welfare policy for the 1990s*. Cambridge: Harvard University Press.

Burtless, G. (1990). *A future of lousy jobs: The changing structure of U.S. wages*. Washington, DC: Brookings Institution.

Center on Budget and Policy Priorities. (1992). Number in poverty hits 20-year high. Washington, DC.

Danziger, S., R. Haveman, and R. Plotnick. (1981). How income transfer programs affect work, savings, and the income distribution: A critical review. *Journal of Economic Literature*, 19.

Elwood, D. (1988). *Poor support*. New York: Basic Books.

Fiedler, E. R. (1989). Economic policies to control stagflation. In C. Lowell-Harris, Ed., Inflation: Long-term problems. *Proceedings of the Academy of Political Science*, 31, 4.

Galbraith, J. K. (1958). *The affluent society*. Boston: Houghton Mifflin.

Gilder, G. (1981). *Wealth and poverty*. New York: Basic Books.

Glazer, N. (1971). The limits of social policy. *Commentary*, 52, 3.

Jencks, C. (1992). *Rethinking social policy: Race, Poverty, and the underclass*. Cambridge: Harvard University Press.

Jencks, C., and K. Edin. (1990). The real welfare problem. *TAP*, No. 1., Spring.

Kaus, M. (1992). *The end of equality*. New York: Basic Books.

Krugman, P. (1990). *The age of diminished expectations: U.S. economy policy in the 1990s*. Cambridge: MIT Press.

Lampman, R. (1979). *Focus* 4, 1. Madison: Institute for Research on Poverty, University of Wisconsin.

Mead, L. M. (1992). *The new politics of poverty: The nonworking poor in America*. New York: Basic Books.

Medoff, J. (April 1992). The new unemployment. Prepared for Senator Lloyd Bentsen, Chairman, Subcommittee on Economic Growth, Trade, and Taxes, Joint Economic Committee, April 1992 (Revised December 4, 1992).

Moynihan, D. P. (1973). *The politics of a guaranteed income: The Nixon administration and the Family Assistance Plan*. New York: Random House.

Moynihan, D. P. (1992). How the Great Society "destroyed the American family." *The Public Interest*.

Phillips, A. W. (1958). The relation between unemployment and the rate of change of money wage rates in the United Kingdom, 1981-1957. *Economica*, 25.

Polanyi, K. (1957). *The great transformation*. Boston: Beacon Press.

Porter, K. H. (March 1990). Making JOBS work: What research says about effective employment programs for AFDC recipients. Center on Budget and Policy Priorities, Washington, DC.

Sasser, J. *The New York Times O-Ed*. February 2, 1993.

Schram, S. F. (1992). Post-positivistic policy analysis and the Family Support Act of 1988: symbols at the expense of substance. *Polity*, 24, 4.

Schwartz, J. E., and T. J. Volgy. (1992) *Forgotten Americans*. New York: W. W. Norton & Co.

Chapter 2

Revisiting the Unseen: Some Unresolved Issues in Homeless Advocacy and Research

Kim Hopper

INTRODUCTION

The Impetus to Rethink

As the homeless relief effort extends well into its second decade, making this the longest period of sustained homelessness in this nation's history, it may be an appropriate time to take stock of some guiding premises. Having done so, it should be clearer to all of us why the theme for this presentation is "the unseen." I want to use the term in two distinct senses. I mean first the myopia that occurs as an occupational hazard in the practical arts of law, ministry, and medicine, to say nothing of social work or, for that matter, anthropology. Whether we speak the language of individual rights, patient needs, private sins, or everyday custom, *knowing well* typically means *knowing small*, within the close confines of one's own field of practice. Doing good for another, William Blake reminds us, means working with "minute particulars." While close focus may enhance craft, it tends to impede analysis: the tight quarters of effective action in the immediate case are not normally the same boundaries that shed light on the origins of the target class or its problems. Much, even the late collateral effects of one's own actions, remains unseen.

In addition to this occupational myopia, there is a second sense in which I apply this term "unseen." I argue that the typical state of provisions for the homeless poor is *institutional invisibility*; further, from a cultural standpoint, I want to suggest that this is no accident.

The impetus to undertake this task of rethinking comes from two directions: my experience as an advocate working to ameliorate homelessness for the last fifteen years, and my reading of the history of prior efforts to address homelessness in places like New York City. Each of these, in turn, convinced me that attempts to tackle homelessness on its own terms risked misreading (and badly so) what the problem was all about. So, my argument will first survey some of the salient limits of advocacy—specifically, *advocacy as special pleading*—as they have taken shape in the last decade or so; then, I will draw upon a historical reading of provisions for homeless men in New York. I want to begin, however, with some observations on a recent book about homeless women, which I think neatly captures the tension between close focus and depth of field.

Making It Homeless

Economists borrow a word from physics, *hysteresis*, to describe the cumulative complexity of a destabilized system, careening from one induced adjustment to another, getting progressively further off course and out of balance, such that restoration to its original state is an ever more costly and difficult affair. One way of highlighting the difficulties that we advocates—and I venture to suggest, social workers—have when it comes to "big picture" issues, is to recall that much of our work takes place in this zone of hysteresis. We are often madly scurrying to mute the damage to lives that seem to be amassing further injury and deeper captivity at every turn. As an ethnographer, too, I feel a particular affinity for this sort of occupational myopia. I am not alone.

Tell Them Who I Am (1993), an extraordinary book by the late Elliot Liebow, may be read as a sustained meditation on hysteresis as it unfolds on the margins of homelessness. In the care it takes to render a scrupulous inventory of these homeless women's lives, this book ranks up there with (another oddly named documentary) *Let Us Now Praise Famous Men* (1941), James Agee and Walker Evans' moving tribute to Alabaman tenant farmers during the Depression. Unlike Agee and Evans, however, Liebow does not describe the exertions of kinsfolk looking after their homesteads but rather the daily lives of a contrived community of women who have none. These women live in the lowest form of what the Census Bureau coyly refers to as "group quarters." About the only thing they have in common (at least when they arrive) is the need for such refuge. Among other things (and perhaps most surprising of all), *Tell Them Who I Am* is about the prospects of sisterhood (Liebow calls it "solidarity") in this most unlikely of settings.[1]

First and foremost, this is a book about toil and trouble. Unlike their beaten-down counterparts of yesteryear, memorialized in such Depression-era accounts as Tom Kromer's *Waiting for Nothing*, and unlike too their skid-row brethren of the 1950s and 1960s, these women (most of them anyhow) are anything but reconciled to their fate. Energy, effort, and resolve make frequent appearances through-out this book—as surely do failure, frustration, and disappointment. As the shelters, the streets, thoughtless passersby, skinflint employ-ers, service providers, and other assorted grifters put these women through their paces, we learn (safely, from afar) to take the measure of their homelessness as a job, not (or only as it entails still *more* work) as a status.

If the *work of homelessness* is this book's real subject, and the portrayal of that work one of its singular achievements, its implied target—and the focus of its recommendations—is the social factory that demands such exertions. For what is at once so moving, sad, and infuriating about the stories told here is that these heroic labors are mustered in the service of so thankless and gratuitous a cause: making do without a place of one's own. Such work, this book makes plain, ultimately counts for very little. With few exceptions (one homeless woman's accumulation of a nest egg), this work returns little on the investment, persuades few people of personal worth, and amasses no equity. Nonetheless, the practice mat-ters—the labor itself not the product—and matters hugely because what is reaped in the process are dividends of a tentative self-regard and, if only in the sharing of stupidities endured, a precarious kind of community.

Now, six out of the seven chapters in the book describe the daily struggles to survive in the shelter or on the street. It is, I suspect, the tension between Kromer's admiration for the arduous work of homelessness as performed by these women and his abhorrence of the conditions that stage and require it that accounts for these uneven proportions of description and prescription in the book.[2] If one *were* to draw a single moral from the terrifically detailed first part of the book, it would be something irked and weary along the lines of the following: *there is no fair measure here.* For these women, like the hypothesized off-kilter system that I began this section with, each day brings new challenges, only rarely muted—let alone advanced—by the exertions that went into surviving the day before. Resolutions of their predicament are not the cumulative product of sustained effort, but a haphazard mix of luck and timing and living long enough to see them. Homelessness is unworthy of the work these women put into its realization; unto labors such as these, more should flow. These are the sort of quasi-biblical pronouncements that come to mind when one completes and reflects upon the first six chapters of Kromer's book.

Liebow's concluding chapter ("Some Thoughts on Homelessness"), however, makes no statements such as those, for the simple and exasperating reason that these observations—faithful though they may be to the ethnography that precedes them—*have nothing to do with solving homelessness.* They are about the practice of homelessness, not its eradication. Instead, and rightly so, Liebow's conclusion takes the form of reflections one could well have arrived at without the painstaking account of toil and trouble that precedes them.[3] (In fact, he wrote them first.) Tellingly, perhaps, they are marked by a summary tone that poorly masks his impatience at having to state the obvious—that affordable housing ("a place of one's own") is in painfully short supply and must be increased; that decent jobs paying living wages are just as necessary; and that for the foreseeable future, we will need shelters characterized by "a minimum of decency and respect" if the gratuitous damage of homelessness is to be reduced. Again, these are observations that can be, and are, regularly made by many whose expertise about the daily tribulations of those homeless is no match for Liebow's.

So the genius of *Tell Them Who I Am* lies not only in its artful documenting of the complexity entailed in surviving as a homeless person, but in its *failure* as a coherent text. Part II—solutions—does not follow from Part I—defensive strategies for surviving while homeless. In that failure, the gap between understanding what it takes to make it homeless and what it might take to eradicate it, lies a small mischievous triumph: by copping out, it tricks the reader into rediscovering, as if for the first time, the simple truth about an ounce of prevention.

Note how easily a kind of occupational blindness might very well have afflicted this book had Liebow remained true to his ethnographic compass: if he had told us what the natives told him, showed us by design what they showed him by inadvertence. What he found to celebrate in the lives of these women—their gritty determination not to give in to the press of circumstance and pull of despair—is worthless as a remedy for homelessness. Worse still, without that awkwardly tacked-on reality-check of a final chapter, his portrayal could well have invited casual readers to romanticize the nobility of the street and its rigors. A more perverse twist to the author's intent is difficult to imagine.

My claim is simple: Advocacy for the homeless poor in the 1980s and early 1990s has too often fallen prey to a similar hazard. Mesmerized by the details, driven by the injustice, and consumed by the job of arresting the damage and protecting the puny gains made, we have managed to let much escape our notice.

THE LIMITS OF SPECIAL PLEADING

I take it that the task before us is to move beyond a reform movement based upon successive ad hoc improvisations, devised under "emergency" decrees, and fashioned for the most part to tackle only the most grievous of hardships. The argument I want to make may be summarized as follows.

The Argument in Brief

If reform is to be broad-based, it must be rooted in a demand for public goods whose benefits will be widely distributed (or appreciated). If so, then demands rooted in "rights talk" are increasingly problematic. The difficulties are ones of both scale and of strategy. Special pleading—the definitive form that advocacy for the homeless took in the 1980s—makes sense when the aggrieved class is small and the sought-after remedies take the form of "reasonable accommodations." This is when reform entails not fundamental changes in the societal mechanisms for the distribution of scarce goods, but adjustments at the margins, such as corrections in sorting mechanisms to make them less biased, or enforcement of agreements long ago reached on paper in the courts and legislatures. When the target class is huge—for affordable housing, according to one recent reckoning, it is "one-third of a nation" (Stone, 1993)—and needed remedies are substantial—potentially, no less than a collective decision to treat the provision of housing as a necessity rather than a commodity—it may be a mistake to opt for a strategy of reform by attrition. And that is precisely what advocates have done: We have multiplied the distinctive warrants by means of which successive subgroups of the homeless poor could claim a "special needs" entitlement to subsidized housing. Each warrant is rooted in a differential inability to purchase housing on the market. From such a perspective, the limits on advocacy are essentially those of the imagination. New varieties of compensable disability await ever more discerning readings of unusual hardship, and ever more clever manipulation of established precedent. Thus, the rolls of recognized disability will proliferate as will entitlement to goods too scarce to be petitioned by appeal to a common need.

In this way, presumably, social justice may be achieved through stealth, by the slow accretion of classes of specially entitled groups. What this amounts to in practice is an endless round of queue jumping, as successive waves of "special needs" populations plead their case to move to the front of the line. What it neglects is politics, in all its guises. The lessons we are learning from prolonged efforts at judicial reform[4]—the defection of supporters put off by the affront to equity that appeals to "exceptions" invariably raise and the bitter fruit of local struggles to wrest control of land uses and property rights—all suggest that such tactics may be short-sighted.

What Prompts Such Reconsideration?

Questions about the strategic choices made by advocates in the 1980s come from four different areas: the portrayal of remedies to homelessness, the definition of the class, the acknowledgment of disability, and the role of government.[5]

Shelter and Housing Have Never Solved Homelessness

The success of efforts to stem homelessness has very little to do with the design of shelters, of their rules of eligibility and occupancy. Demand for shelter is defined by default. It is a function of labor market, cheap housing, welfare regulations and benefit levels, police practices and commitment policies and practices, and the tolerance and support capacity of kin. True, targeted housing can claim some successes. It resolved the New York City homeless family crises of 1948-1949 and 1973; it has relocated thousands of homeless families in recent years. I do not mean to gainsay such accomplishments. In retrospect, however, these were largely the illusory gains of queue jumping, e.g., privileging homeless families' applications for public housing at the expense of others.

Incremental demands for housing as a solution to homelessness are vulnerable on a number of fronts.

1. Housing alone will not suffice for many; supports will be necessary to ensure stability because there is no excess capacity to accommodate the mobility that previously enabled the occasionally disruptive or troublesome tenant to "maintain housing" in the private market. In the past, such people simply moved around a lot. That is no longer an option today, and attention must shift to the contextual factors that stabilize residency.

2. The very success of the remedies achieved through special pleading has provoked some unintended consequences that threaten to erode the political consensus which made privileged access possible in the first place. Numerous problems have arisen both because of the nature of some of the accompanying problems and the bureaucratic snags in implementation. The specific problem I have in mind is the affront to equity and sense of fairness that may arise when shelters are thought to function as triage mechanisms. Note that the objection targets *not* legitimate need but its presumed proxy—the declaration of oneself as officially homeless and the concomitant willingness

to endure the modern means test of waiting in temporary quarters for a "placement." These have become the new, suspect rule of exceptionalism.

3. Finally, to speak simply of "affordability" begs the question of livelihood: What are such people to do after they awake in the morning, having moved from being privileged homeless to merely poor. Disenchantment occurs when the approach is simply to reduce rents. So, for example, one may reap certain efficiencies of project-based assistance by lumping needy tenants together in large numbers, but only at the cost of the stability that a more integrated tenancy would bring.

The Homeless Poor Are Not a Discrete Class of the Indigent

Standing patterns of residential instability are the rule. It is the failure of routine makeshifts, not distinctive traits or markers of difference, that appears to matter most. This is especially clear if we look at shelter use over time. Three percent of the population of Philadelphia and New York City made use of public shelters in three and five years, respectively, in the early 1990s (Culhane et al., 1994).

At the same time, advocates have reluctantly learned that to ignore the evidence of difference and disability is both to lose credibility and to cede the argument to others.[6]

Paying Attention to Disabilities Need Not Mean "Blaming the Victim"

It is indisputable that certain disabilities put people at enhanced risk of displacement and handicap their chances of exiting from homelessness. Just like race, gender, and other coded differences (Minow 1992), these risks are rooted in relations to others and to markets; they do not, in some essential sense, *inhere* in the people themselves. Put differently, it is not disability per se, but its social and practical meaning—the difference it makes in specific settings and time—that is consequential. I have in mind such things as its effects on the support capacity of kin, its ability to exploit (in bygone days) the accommodating tendencies of "disreputable" housing (Groth, 1983) where excess vacancy could invariably be found, and its status as a legitimate and protected condition (Stone, 1984).

Government's Role in Subsidizing Housing Is Likely to Change

Owing to substantial changes in labor and housing markets, at least for the interim, government (or government in partnership with for-profit and not-for-profit agents) will have to do with deliberation and planning what the market once achieved through profiteering, inefficiency, and slack or absent oversight. The government must look for ways of re-creating or supporting those marginal resources—spot work, substandard housing, erratic income, more viable kin, and other activities grouped in the informal economy. The margins have dramatically shrunken, where they have not disappeared altogether, and deliberate work will be needed to re-create the rude shelter, lousy jobs and rough tolerance traditionally found there. Government will need to find new ways to indirectly increase housing capacity, shore up the support capacity of kin, and increase demand for productive activities intended for use not for trade.

Abeyance: An Alternative Framework

The makeshift character so evident in contemporary relief efforts proves to be a sturdy motif in the public response to the homeless poor. Well into the Great Depression, when the legitimacy of need would seem to have been self-evident, local homeless relief efforts were distinguished by their ad hoc, even haphazard character. That the same observation applies today, a decade and a half into this latest resurgence of official homelessness, suggests that some deeper template of response may be at work. Both periods saw profound changes in livelihood coupled with major shifts in the social mechanisms—formal and informal—for handling excess (and potentially troublesome) populations. A useful way of framing the larger problem, of which literal homelessness is only a fragment, is provided by the notion of the "abeyance process" (Mizruchi, 1987; Hopper and Baumohl, 1994).

"Abeyance" refers to the recurring problem of a mismatch between the available positions in a society (too few) and the supply of potential claimants to those positions (too many). Various mechanisms, devised under a host of nonmarket auspices, have been resorted to in order to produce supplemental "status slots" to absorb surplus adults of laboring age. Whether it was the state (frontier settlements, public works, compulsory education), the church (monasteries, breakaway religious orders), or even countercultural strains (communal experiments, intentional communities), *such measures provided livelihood and, if necessary, housing for "redundant" people who might otherwise have posed a disruptive threat to social order.* In the postfeudal world, they did so by supplying virtual work that was "materially uncompetitive with participation in main-line economic activities" (Mizruchi, 1987: 157). In market economies, they function effectively as human warehouses, "hold[ing] personnel out of the labor force at a cost that contributes to the maintenance of low wages in the economic sphere" (Mizruchi, 1987: 157-158).

It takes little imagination to see how contemporary shelters fill precisely this function, albeit uneasily, for at least some of the homeless poor (their most obvious defect, one lamented since the turn of the century, is their failure to provide useful work). Shelters, from this perspective, should be seen as site-specific, partial solutions to the more general problem—not of housing—but of unemployment. In much the same way as official unemployment figures are a poor guide to the severity and depth of joblessness, official homelessness can be seen as a pale and untrustworthy index of residential instability. And, as labor-market analysts have learned to examine alternative "employments" in military service, prisons, hospitals, and the informal economy (Moss and Tilly, 1991), so historians of official homelessness will have to take account of the absorptive capacities of nonhomeless institutions and informal practices (such as "doubling up"). Much as those same economists fret over the disincentives to waged work posed by such alternative employments, this analysis should shed some light on what some anthropologists call the "institution effect"[7]—namely, the moral hazard created by such structures as shelters when viewed as viable alternatives to work, rent payment, and troublesome kin.

Simply, interest in abeyance prompts us to ask what redundant people will *do* once the sun is up, not merely where they will sleep at night. This concern links in principle the domains of labor and housing, raising anew the issue of how homelessness should be classified as a "social problem." Properly instituted, abeyance practices not only "warehouse" redundant people (usually in surplus structures), but engage otherwise idle hands. If even monks performing surrogate penances for "sinner[s] who could afford the price" may be considered to be at work, doing "jobs, particularly the kind that required no special talent" (Mizruchi, 1987: 33), then it could be argued that solutions to redundancy that fail to make such a provision will be faulty, unstable, and prone to unravel. I want to suggest that that is precisely what has happened.

A LEGACY OF DISREGARD

If such matters were typically "unseen" by advocates in the trenches, theirs was by no means the only blindness. What is noteworthy about homeless relief efforts over time is not only their ad hoc, makeshift character, but the cloak of disregard that conventionally surrounds their operation.

The Argument from Anthropology and History

Reviewing the record of the state's attempts to address homelessness, one is impressed by the consistent pattern of official deferral. If there is one thing that characterizes homeless relief policy, it is improvisation: the steady production of measures designed to cope with a declared "crisis" while forestalling—indeed, typically denying the need for—any lasting institutional reform. The history of New York City's sheltering efforts is illustrative. "Outbreaks" of homelessness (the epidemiological trope is unavoidable) are ignored for as long as possible, shunted whenever practicable to penal or custodial alternatives, referred to private charity, and—when all other options have been exhausted—faced directly, albeit (in the words of one of its abler chroniclers, Nels Anderson) "in the easiest and most expedient manner" (1934: 1). So long as homelessness can be framed as a temporary aberration, the fiction can be maintained that nothing more serious than deranged minds, bad habits, or faulty coping skills is at stake.

As a hybrid branch of poor relief—part "indoor" and confined, part "outdoor" and dispersed—most of the operations of public shelter take place in deep shadows, an ironic echo of the erstwhile labor of its occupants.

Historically, that is, the work done by otherwise homeless men when employed—laying track; digging tunnels, mines, ditches, and canals; cutting timber; roughnecking on oil rigs; harvesting crops—is "dirty work." Low wages, risky work, abysmal living conditions, and the uncertain terms of the contract make such work the lowest sort of employment. I want to propose that such labor has its institutional counterpart in the public work of providing shelter. Consider the following: Facilities for the management and support of marginal people operate for the most part without the distraction of outside scrutiny.[8] A kind of tacit agreement appears to have been struck with the public *not* to look too closely at how public lodging for indigents actually works. Typically, some obscure backwater bureaucracy is given the job ("the Siberia of HRA" [the welfare department] was how the Men's Shelter was referred to in New York City). Even when crisis hits—new reports of street homelessness in New York City antedated the filing of *Callahan* by nearly a decade—the public's first response is to seek reassurance that corrective measures are in place, competent administration is on the case, and evidence of progress is soon to be at hand.

Not only to its charges but to the work itself, then, the old adage applied: out of sight, out of mind.

Inevitably, there is anthropology that illustrates this pattern. I refer specifically to what anthropologists in recent years have taken to calling the "work of culture"—that set of symbols and social practices whose "job" it is to channel painful, potentially disruptive feelings into publicly sanctioned forms of expression. In this way, for example, the grief of bereavement is given voice and form through collective, ritualized vehicles of mourning. If custom and belief can be put to the service of expression, might not social practice be bent in the contrary, indeed, opposite direction as well—as vehicles of repression, of habitual *un*awareness? A number of authors have argued so (Hughes 1963; Coser 1969; Feldman 1994), and it strikes me that a case may be made that public shelter routinely operates in precisely this fashion.

With respect to the dirty work of shelter, then, how does it happen that so much of it goes on without occasioning the slightest interest on the part of the host populace? Two means have traditionally been employed.

The first, which has received a good deal of commentary in recent years, is to cast target populations in the mold of deviance. Vagrancy in the nineteenth century was fundamentally a question of character: tramps were a moral scourge and a subversive subculture; nomadism, a psychiatric disorder; and skid row, the last refuge of derelicts.[9] In such a world, shelter becomes a necessary modality of containment, a way of protecting the public against the threat of dangerous others. There are signs that in the eyes of some at least, this world still thrives today:

- A *New York Times* editorial written ten years ago railed against the presence of street people who "continue to consume tax dollars and demoralize society" (April 9, 1984).
- Six years later, Myron Magnet opined in an op-ed piece that "what you see if you stop to look, is craziness, drunkenness, dope, and danger . . . the homeless are an encyclopedia of social pathology and mental disorder" (1990).
- In a book hailed by *Wall Street Journal* reviewers, Bill Bradley and Andrew Cuomo, Baum and Burnes argued that once the veil of "denial" is yanked down, it will be plain that homeless people *may be defined* as those "whose ability to function in ordinary social and economic interactions has been so impaired by their disabling conditions [mental illness and substance abuse especially] that they are socially alienated from their various support networks and society's institutions and are unable to maintain an independent living" (1993: 119).
- More recently still, of course, tuberculosis and HIV infection have been added to the roster of pathology. In September 1993, Pete Hamill called for the forced confinement of street dwellers who refuse the invitation to return for retooling to "homeless sanctuaries"—a modern place of "wholesome penitentiary" (citation), where, as "menaces to public health," they will be treated for their additions, put through a therapeutic boot camp, educated for employment, and for good measure, exposed to the classics. Those too disabled to graduate would be "returned to the institutions" from whence they decamped in the first place and where they properly ought to reside.

It would be a mistake to dismiss such recommendations as the wailings of a few cranks. The lesson they mean to teach is plain: homeless people constitute not merely a symbolic token of "disorder,"[10] but a literal plague. If not a "quarantine" (as Hamill urges), then at least a sound containment policy is in order. Shelter becomes a logical extension of police power; the architecture of disease control should be its guiding logic.

There is a second means of deflecting notice, one that sounds a similar theme but in a subtler fashion. This time the moral question of confinement is not to be justified by appeal to an epidemiological warrant, as it disposed of altogether, by the simple expedient of treating homelessness as a *routine* problem of municipal sanitation. The disposition of surplus—unneeded people who can claim no proper place of their own—is seen as a simple problem of waste disposal. Like its physical counterpart, this is best viewed as an exacting but humdrum job, best left to specialists. Specialized departments (the "Shelter Care Center for Men"), staffed by trained personnel (caseworkers, institutional aides), operating for the most part under the cover of night and well off the beaten path comprise the machinery that will see to it that appropriate action is taken, rest assured, the details of which need not concern the rest of us. Should a moment's query afflict an unusually inquisitive citizen, he or she might reflect that the very invisibility of such work may be taken as proof positive of its effectiveness.

In either interpretation, public lodging of the indigent joins a number of other distasteful chores performed by the modern state. Generically, to them falls the task (as John Stuart Mill put it long ago) of quelling "the spectacle of pain" and, preferably, removing it from public view altogether. Others have elaborated the argument. C. Everett Hughes (1962) suggests that we extend "a kind of unconscious mandate" to those designated functionaries who do "the dirty work of society"—acting out "impulses of which we are or wish to be less aware." Lewis Coser (1969) adds that the structural contingency that makes this displacement possible is "relative lack of visibility." Most recently, Alan Feldman has invited us to examine how our perceptual apparatus itself is manipulated in the service of a cultivated "cultural amnesia" (1994).

Thus does culture domesticate cruelty, necessary and otherwise, by assigning the job of afflicting it to unseen agents, whose work is surveilled (if at all) by invisible monitors, and whose records are kept in anticipation of (the unlikely event of) having to render a justifiable "account" of themselves (Garfinkel, 1967). It is only when gratuitous suffering escapes its assigned keep, when it intrudes insistently in the daily lives of ordinary people—when, in the language introduced earlier, abeyance fails and the safely excluded wander off the reservation—it is only then that the "visibility of evil" (Coser's terms) thrusts itself back into the sphere of sanctioned inspection. Only then—in an act normally accompanied by a gasp of surprise, even incredulity, by the keepers—is what had been a collective policy of disregard opened anew for examination. The unraveling of normal abeyance processes and their massive failure in some cases—Jim Baumohl and I have argued elsewhere (1994)—is what happened to homelessness in the 1980s.

Abeyance: Some Implications for Advocacy

So what does all this mean for reworking the agenda of advocacy? I can think of five areas that are ripe for rethinking and where rather immediate implications are discernible.[11]

Relations with the Public

Public attitudes toward homelessness, the survey researchers tell us, are both ill-formed and full of internal tensions. Advocates would do well to take seriously the job of presenting the picture of homelessness in all its complexity. Despite reams of anecdotal evidence of a reputedly hostile public, it is not as though we have the makings of a plebiscite on the issue. Most reports of outraged citizenry concern opposition to local proposals that engage a host of issues not specific to this target population (Piller 1991). Nor is it the case that success stores—What works in rehousing folks? For whom? Under what circumstances? At what costs?—have been widely circulated. Curiously, when something "works" in rehousing, it tends to vacate the homeless policy premises altogether, preferring the invisibility of "neighbor" to the showcase status of "formerly homeless."

Housing

With respect to housing—and especially with respect to housing as a social good and not just a market commodity—advocates will need to tighten the logic of demands and explore their fiscal feasibility and implications for larger questions of equity. In particular, they must argue convincingly that, for some needy groups at least, support services perform the same functional role as debt service, insulation, and emergency fire exits: They make that housing habitable. On a more ambitious front, the case for expanding "social ownership" of housing—dwellings traded outside the private speculative market—will need to be bolstered. The definitive feature of such housing is that its occupants, while not technically owners, enjoy all the privileges of secure tenure except the right to sell or bequeath the property. Debt service could be reduced through federal grants; profit would be eliminated; a range of takeover options could be considered. A great deal of groundwork has been laid (Stone, 1993: 191-217), but cultural barriers (a "home" is the closest thing most families will ever have to a substantial bequest), not to mention stiff opposition from the lending industry, make the pursuit of intermediate steps in the direction of social ownership (union-owned housing, limited-equity cooperatives with severe resale restrictions, land trusts, etc.) all the more important as object lessons.

The Antinomies of Work

Nothing is bound to raise more red flags, excite memories of a (purportedly) failed history, or throw the usual lines of political allegiance into confusion than the prospect of large-scale public-sector employment. If the preceding analysis has any claim to merit, useful work for those otherwise "idle" is an inescapable subject. Not that the conceptual issues are settled (What activities, at home or not, should count as "useful work"?), the political ground cleared of obstacles,[12] or popular confusion dispelled (the difference between workfare and work relief, to mention just one persisting misunderstanding). Nor have recent attempts to rehabilitate the political relevance of public job creation—the hyperbolic character of the most extensively argued case for work in recent days (Kaus, 1992), the appropriation of makework by an increasingly punitive discourse on welfare reform, the proposal by a serious social scientist that homeless people be offered a flophouse room in exchange for four hours of work a day (Jencks, 1994)—helped to clarify matters. More consequential is the transformation of the world at work at large (e.g., *Business Week* XX, October 1994), especially the growth of a large corps of "contingent" (part-time) workers; developments such as these make the lot of those on the margins of the labor market something less than pressing (see *The New York Times*, October 23, 1994: 22).

Still, if the argument offered here has a gravitational center, it is that *credible forms of useful activity*—socially valued work or its equivalents—are essential to the successful reenfranchisement of those redundant to the market's needs. The argument extends to many of those disabled by severe mental illness as well (Warner 1994). If contemporary appeals to a rewritten "social contract" are to have practical merit, real opportunities—not rancorous slogans—are needed. Not only do a myriad projects suggest themselves, ranging from provision of day care to repair of infrastructure, but a side benefit would be reaped as well: This culture has invariably proved more tolerant of those who have, one way or another, *earned* their vices.

The Issue of Race

Few issues were more effectively buried in the past decade of homeless commentary and advocacy than that of race. This remains the case despite persisting evidence that, in a decisive break with the issue's past, minorities are regularly overrepresented in studies of homeless persons today (Shlay and Rossi, 1992; Hopper, 1996). No doubt, the absence of color from contemporary debates on homeless policy owes much to a strategic decision, made early on by advocates, to stress the "just like us" character of the homeless poor in an effort to build public sympathy (White, 1990-1991). It should be clear by now that whatever the gain in short-run compassion, a price was paid in implicit racism. For all its avowed commitment to "larger linkages," the discourse on homelessness, like much of the poverty debate at large, seemed content to banish the race question to the well-fenced confines of "the underclass" (Katz, 1993). In the process, it reproduced the same marginalization its champions had decried.

Culture and Representation

Finally, if one crucial lesson has been learned of late in advocacy circles, it is that *speaking for* homeless people—especially when it comes to "tell[ing] them who I am" (Liebow, 1993)—must give way to collaborative efforts to render plainly both the realities of homelessness and the feasibility of solutions. Such efforts remain scarce, even as calls for making them have intensified. Relatedly, as behavior ("dependency") has become the leitmotif of welfare positions on the Right, "culture" has reappeared (after a 20-year absence) as its enabling matrix. Nowhere is this clearer than in neoconversative analyses of poverty (Butler and Kondratas, 1987), especially African-American poverty (Mead, 1992). While few would argue that culture plays no role in sustaining putatively self-destructive patterns of behavior, it is by no means clear that *distinctive* subcultures (even if one allows, for argument's sake, the beliefs, values, and practices in question) are at work (Hochschild, 1991; Nightingale, 1993). The broader point, as Wilson argued some time ago (1987), is that "culture" cannot long be ignored without reappearing as a wild-card variable in the hands of opponents, the more dangerous for having escaped examination. Advocates would do well to heed the warning.

CONCLUSION: QUEUING FOR JUSTICE?

. . . waiting may also be costly in itself, notwithstanding the value of foregone alternatives. This latter tendency deserves more attention than it has received. (Schwartz, 1975: 167)

In confronting the unseen, the first step is choosing, deliberately, to look. The second is to begin grappling honestly with the complexities that stand newly revealed upon reexamination. The fundamental claim of this argument may be stated simply: When it comes to affordable housing, and especially when that involves public subsidies, the decision rules that make for orderly queues and the appearance of fairness—while at the same time recognizing and making allowances for urgency of need—are in a shambles. This is a bit more encompassing a claim than those that usually issue from sustained examinations of homelessness, and a closing word in its defense may be in order. To do so, let me use an example closer at hand that illustrates the same principle.

I refer to the growing and much-maligned practice of poor people "misusing" emergency rooms as their preferred primary care provider. After two decades during which the notion of a "health care crisis" moved from the margins of political discourse to its centerpiece (at least for a while), we have learned to take the measure of such practices as something other than ignorance, irrationality, or a subcultural impatience with waiting one's turn. For health care planning purposes, misuse of emergency rooms joins a host of other "sentinel events"—the original roster included "all unnecessary diseases, disabilities and untimely deaths"—devised by epidemiologists as a composite measure of the quality of general medical care and public health (Rutstein et al., 1976). If heeded, such anomalies may serve as an early warning system signaling deficiencies and/or gaps in the current health service system. More to the point here, such a framework suggests that this particular practice should be read for something other than its face value—not as reason to further rationalize and tighten triaging procedures at the ER, but as a warrant to examine the inadequacies of alternative sources of care, obstacles to access, and the costs of using them.

No less than that is required, I have tried to show, when it comes to rethinking current homelessness policy. I do not want to diminish the difficulties involved in doing so, but neither do I wish to downplay my own conviction that we really have no other choice.

NOTES

1. Especially unanticipated, in this respect, is the humor in this book, especially the keen eye these women have for absurdity and pretense—of which, in the world of homeless relief, there is plenty. My favorite is Kim's being told that she would have to "provide proof of no income" (p. 142), followed by Peggy's "contract" according to which she agreed "not to try to kill myself for two weeks" (p. 130), and by the social worker's response to Michelle's "distraught" worries at the prospect of the Refuge closing: "The answer, you'll find, is within *you*" (p. 134).

2. Liebow's own explanation is less structural: "I ran out of gas"; he found himself too fatigued to do the necessary work (remarks at the American Sociological Association session on the book, Los Angeles, August 2, 1994).

3. Others have done so—because such matters go to the root of social security, broadly understood, in the United States today.

4. Regarding the Willowbrook Wars (Rothman and Rothman 1984), for example, Martha Minow (1992) has commented: "The more powerfully legal claims on behalf of [aggrieved groups] push for change at the deeper, structural level, the more likely are there to be objections, from many quarters, to their use of law to reform society" (p. 367).

5. These are spelled out in much greater detail in Hopper and Baumohl, 1994:522-552.

6. As W. J. Wilson (1987) has remarked, this also occurred to studies of the African-American family in the wake of the culture of poverty debates.

7. This is more generic version of what Western economists refer to as Say's Law, with the addition of a cultural gloss. With respect to inpatient treatment of clinical depression in Sri Lanka, for example, Obeyeskere writes: "If the institution did not exist, people might be compelled by their kinship obligations to accommodate these patients in their own homes, and this in turn would inevitably lead to the conceptualization of the depressive affects in Buddhist existential terms" (p. 149).

8. Note that the surrender of a "liberty interest" which earns institutional inmates—at least in principle—additional rights as well as much closer supervision of the conditions of their confinement does not apply here.

9. For further discussion of the historical evidence on this point, see Hopper (1991).

10. See Kelling (1990) and Wilson (1987) on "broken window" theory (citation).

11. Again, the more complete version may be found in Hopper and Baumohl 1994.

12. See Levitan and Gallo (1992) for a review.

REFERENCES

Agee, J., and Evans, W. (1941). *Now let us praise famous men*. New York: Harper.

Anderson, N. (1934). *The homeless of New York*. New York: Welfare Council.

Baum, A. S., and Burnes, D. W. (1993). *A nation in denial*. Boulder: Westview.

Business Week (October 17, 1994). Special Issue on "Rethinking Work."

Butler, S., and Kondratas, S. A. (1987). *Out of the poverty trap*. New York: Free Press.

Coser, L. A. (1969). The visibility of evil. *Journal of Social Issues* 25: 101-109.

Culhane, D. P., Dejowski, E. F., Ibanez, J., Nedham, E., and Macchia, I. (1994). Public shelter admission rates in Philadelphia and New York City. *Housing Policy Debate* 5: 107-140.

Feldman, A. (1994). On cultural amnesia. *American Ethnologist* 21: 404-418.

Garfinkel, H. (1967). *Studies in ethnomethodology.* Englewood-Cliffs, NJ: Prentice-Hall.

Groth, P. (1983). Forbidden housing. PhD Dissertation. Berkeley: University of California-Berkeley.

Hamill, P. (September 20, 1993). How to save the homeless and ourselves. *New York Magazine.*

Hochschild, J. (1991). The politics of the estranged poor. *Ethics* 101: 560-578.

Hopper, K. (1991). A poor apart: The distancing of homeless men in New York's history. *Social Research* 58: 107-3134.

Hopper, K. (1996). Margins within margins: Homelessness among African-American Men. In S. C. Nolutshungu (ed.), *Margins of Insecurity: Minorities and International Security.* Rochester: University of Rochester Press, pp. 213-249.

Hopper, K., and Baumohl, J. (1994). Held in abeyance: Rethinking homelessness and advocacy. *American Behavioral Scientist* 37: 522-552.

Hughes, C. E. (1962). Good people and dirty work. *Social Problems* 10: 3-11.

Katz, M. B. (1993). The urban "underclass" as a metaphor of social transformation. In M. B. Katz (ed.), *The "underclass" debate.* Princeton, NJ: Princeton University Press, pp. 3-23.

Kaus, M. (1992). *The end of equality.* New York: Basic Books.

Kelling, G. (1990). Affidavit to New York State Supreme Court on behalf of defendants in *Wally versus New York Transit Authority.*

Kromer, T. (1935). *Waiting for nothing.* New York: Alfred Knopf.

Levitan, S., and Gallo, F. (1992). *Spending to save.* Washington, DC: George Washington University.

Liebow, E. (1993). *Tell them who I am.* New York: Basic Books.

Magnet, M. (1990). Homeless: Craziness, dope, and danger. *The New York Times,* January 26.

Mead, L. (1992). *The new politics of poverty.* New York: Basic Books.

Mill, J. S. (1962). Civilization. In G. Himmelfarb (ed.), *Essays on politics and culture.* New York: Doubleday.

Minow, M. (1992). *Making all the difference.* Ithaca, NY: Cornell University Press.

Mizruchi, E. (1987). *Regulating society,* second edition. Chicago: University of Chicago Press.

Moss, P., and Tilly, C. (1991). *Why black men are doing worse in the labor market.* New York: Social Science Research Council.

Nightingale, C. H. (1993). *On the edge.* New York: Basic Books.

Obeyeskere, G. (1985). Depression, Buddhism, and the work of culture in Sri Lanka. In A. Kleinman and B. Good (eds.), *Depression and culture.* Berkeley: University of California Press.

Piller, C. (1991). *The fail-safe society.* New York: Basic Books.

Rothman, D. J., and Rothman, S. M. (1984). *The willowbrook wars.* New York: Harper and Row.

Rutstein, D. D., Berenberg, W., Chalmers, T. C., Child, C. G., Fishman, A. P., and Perrin, F. B. (1976). "Measuring the quality of medical care," *New England Journal of Medicine 294*(11): 582-587.

Schwartz, B. (1975). *Queuing and waiting*. Chicago: University of Chicago Press.

Shlay, A. B., and Rossi, P. (1992). Social science research and contemporary studies of homelessness. *Annual Review of Sociology* 18: 129-160.

Stone, D. (1984). *The disabled state*. Philadelphia: Temple University Press.

Stone, M. (1990). *One-third of a nation*. Washington, DC: Economic Policy Institute.

Stone, M. (1993). *Shelter poverty*. Philadelphia: Temple University Press.

Warner, R. (1994). *Recovery from schizophrenia*. Rev. ed. New York: Routledge.

Weir, M. (1992). *Politics and jobs*. Princeton: Princeton University Press.

White, L. (1990-1991). *Representing "The real deal," University of Miami Law Review* 45: 271-313.

Wilson, W. J. (1987). *The truly disadvantaged*. Chicago: University of Chicago Press.

Chapter 3

The Crisis in American Child Welfare

David Fanshel

INTRODUCTION

Spectacular victories were achieved by conservative Republican candidates across the country in November, 1994. The results of this election had powerful implications for the delivery of child welfare services for families and children. In a political environment that presents "tax and spend" as the core of the country's problems, social programs designed to serve the poor will surely be targeted for drastic funding cuts. What might constitute the basic underpinnings of professional social work's approach to the social problems that the election has highlighted? Our coming together today provides an opportunity to exchange views about the controversies that surround us in this time of change.

I assume that I have been invited to participate in this lecture series because I have made a number of research contributions to the child welfare literature dealing with foster care, adoption, preventive services, and protective services. One does not normally think of the empirical researcher whose writings are replete with statistical tables as investing in the larger macro issues of social policy.

A question that holds interest for me is the following: "What research findings coming from the many child welfare research grants you have received, and labors associated with them, do you feel have substance, i.e., represent a significant contribution to the knowledge base of social work?" Put another way: "Is there a substantive social yield from the investment of resources and human creative effort?" This is a question that has significance on a personal as well as a social level. For the former, it relates to one's sense of the worthiness of one's investment of self over many years. To what purpose? This is not a trivial question one faces after retirement. For the latter, the question causes consideration about one's profession and requires a judgment as to whether its members take seriously the task of building the knowledge base that guides practice.

I recently probed the question by scanning the horizon at the contributions of colleagues over the years in a variety of areas of interest to social workers. I was a bit taken aback when I thought of those with distinguished reputations who I could not associate with substantive contributions that had found place in my consciousness. These colleagues seemed to go from one project to another studying diverse subject matter. Often the findings were not clearly defined for the profession and easily forgotten. A project report would be placed on a shelf and the researcher would wait for the next Request for Proposal (RFP) from Washington, DC or the state funding agencies. It was hard to find a social commitment that guided the research effort.

Yet, there was work by others whose findings struck me as evocative, as showing potential applications for practice and/or policy. For example, I thought of Howard Polsky's classic study *Cottage Six* as having interested me in the 1960s because it showed that a children's residential treatment center could invest its resources in individualized psychotherapeutic treatment of its youthful residents while allowing a coercive condition to exist in the cottages where the children lived.[1] Aggressive boys were permitted to bully weaker ones with the seeming connivance of the cottage parents. I know that the finding shook up professionals working in residential care for disturbed children.[2]

In a more recent period, I found of considerable interest the determination that the nature of prenatal care of mothers of infants placed in foster care in New York City was strongly associated with the length of time children remain in care. Using data secured from state health agency sources about individual births, Wulczyn found that prenatal care at any time during pregnancy was associated with lower foster-care placement stays than children born to mothers without the benefit of prenatal care. It was also determined that an increase in the number of low birth-weight infants coming into care, a phenomenon associated with the crack epidemic in New York City, was an important factor in length of time in care. This suggested that healthy babies tend to spend less time in foster care.[3]

My own career has reflected a continuous research interest in the effects of out-of-home placement of children, of the consequences of abuse and neglect for many children who do not leave their homes, and the vulnerabilities of poor families who are the recipients of child welfare preventive services. I am known for rather massive data-gathering studies that look at the life-course development of children as reflected in longitudinal investigations and in follow-up studies exploring their adjustment in adulthood. The research has caused me to ponder the attachment of children to parents even when the latter suffer from dysfunctional characteristics. Thus, when I hear of policy proposals that would consign children to orphanages or that would summarily cut off income support to poor mothers, I have very visceral reactions based upon vivid images of the pain caused children when their families fall apart. The images come from thousands of individual cases probed in great detail in many studies. Over the years, I have been gratified to find validation for most of my views from practitioners whose rich clinical experience has led them to quite similar perspectives about vulnerable children and their families.

I will focus here upon the risks I perceive in the various proposals to change the welfare system. They are mainly from conservative political quarters but are also embraced by those who might be considered moderately liberal.

HOW CHILDREN VIEW THEIR WELFARE MOMS

The emotional needs of poor children are being viewed by radical reformers from the wrong end of the binoculars. Underlying the discourse concerning the topics of "welfare reform" and "family values" is the assumption that the effort to change our social policies in these areas addresses the basic needs of children in the United States. When cavalier proposals are made that would consign children to orphanages, it reveals that the children's welfare is not even being considered because the anger directed at their wayward parents is so intense. Polls have shown, however, that most Americans would balk at harming children.

Children do not have the option of selecting their birth parents. Some are fortunate in being born to fathers and mothers with solid marriages, secure economic circumstances, and under conditions in which family members are relatively free of personal and social handicaps. Other children are the offspring of mothers denied the commitment of a male who acknowledges paternity or who, despite the presence of an identified father, find themselves lacking in paternal financial and emotional support. These mothers are obviously crucial figures in the lives of their offspring and no social program can replace their labors except in the most modest ways.

It is necessary to remind ourselves that the plethora of speeches employing the most derogatory descriptions of "welfare moms" is apt to come to the notice of the children. It may well be an upsetting experience for them. We can say that most of the children born to the women who are not crack addicts, or are otherwise enmeshed in extreme behavioral pathology, develop attachments to their mothers. Having no prior history, a child born under socially disadvantaged circumstances lacks awareness that the woman who is offering maternal care is someone who many believe is worthy of scorn. She is the person who offers milk from her breasts. In the period of early infant development, she changes the baby's diapers, provides clothing and warmth, and protects the baby from harm. The mother is the primary source of affection and stimulation. Such maternal response has a strong hereditary basis in the survival of species, not only among humans.

DENYING HOUSING
TO MOTHERS WITH NEWBORNS

One of the ideas that is gaining favor in the public discourse about welfare reform is the proposal to deny a young mother giving birth to her first child the means to establish an independent household in which she might rear her offspring. President Clinton picked up on this theme in his first State of the Union Address:

This year I will send you a comprehensive welfare reform bill that builds upon the Family Support Act of 1988 and restores the basic values of responsibility. We'll say to teenagers, if you have a child out of wedlock, we will no longer give you a check to set up a separate household. We want families to stay together . . .

The same idea was enunciated earlier by Irving Kristol in his proposal for "A Conservative Welfare State" (*The Wall Street Journal,* June 14, 1993):

These girls should be made to look upon welfare not as an opportunity, but as a frightening possibility. It follows that they should receive no housing allowance—this is probably the most important change of all. Having your own apartment, in which you can raise your child, can be seen as "fun." Living with your child in your parent's home is a lot less alluring.

President Clinton and Mr. Kristol—strange bedfellows given the many differences in their overall social orientations—urge a policy that smacks of a surgical strike against the mother as related to housing. It is not clear how we can summarily deprive the mother of adequate housing while not also potentially creating a grim physical environment for the child. In a study of 160 poor families on the lower east side of New York, our Columbia University research team saw evidence that crowding and associated irritated family relationships often impacted adversely upon children and was correlated with the phenomenon of older youngsters moving into antisocial behavioral patterns.[4]

CUTTING OFF INCOME SUPPORT FROM STRESSED-OUT PARENTS

The number of U.S. children under age six living in poverty experienced a staggering increase between 1987 and 1992—from five to six million—reflecting an all-time high poverty rate of 26 percent for this vulnerable age group, according to a recent report by the National Center for Children in Poverty at Columbia University.[5] Professionals at the center have indicated that the two-decade trend is having devastating consequences on young children today whether they are toddlers or adolescents. The costs of these poverty rates will be paid for over the next two decades.

At recent hearings of the House Ways and Means Committee considering welfare reform, Republican members of Congress affirmed their desire to pass legislation that would cut off cash assistance to unmarried mothers under age 18 whose children are born out of wedlock. They were joined by William J. Bennett, the former Education Secretary who suggested that some states should try cutting off welfare payments for unmarried, teenage mothers: "You actually would see fewer children born out of wedlock. You would see less misery and you could break the cycle of poverty."[6]

Those who seek draconian changes in the provision of income maintenance to the poor rarely talk about what will happen to the children whose mothers are targeted for the harsh penalties being considered. For example, a number of states are enforcing policies whereby a mother who receives financial assistance from the Aid to Families With Dependent Children (AFDC) will be denied budgetary adjustments normally provided in such families when the mother gives birth to another child. There is no consideration whether the newly arrived offspring will be stigmatized within the family and the community as less worthy than the older sibling, and consequently less valued. There is clearly a danger that many of the mothers will develop feelings toward their infants that reflect the influence of the new policy. That is, they will incorporate the sense of shame that is intended by the policy. Do we wish this to happen?

From the experience of studying poor families known to the Lower East Side Family Union in New York City, I and my colleagues, Stephen Finch and John Grundy, gained respect for their valiant efforts to serve their children in the face of difficult personal and social conditions.[7]

Most of the women using AFDC to keep their families together should be seen as representing a very valuable asset to be protected and supported. Their labors come very cheap. As a long-time observer of women who hold their families together under conditions of adversity, I am persuaded of the validity of the truism that nobody will put themselves out for a child like a parent. Their foster care replacement costs are enormous and such replacement is against our avowed national policy.

Clearly, initiatives intended to improve the lives of women on welfare are needed—for their own sakes as well as out of our concern for their children. Social workers who have daily contact with distressed families living in areas of urban blight would see many potential benefits in a policy initiative that offers well-conceived and well-executed training and work opportunities for single mothers. Such activity might liberate them from the stresses and loneliness of confinement to depressing living quarters. These women have been shortchanged all of their lives and deserve a chance for self-betterment. Most certainly their children will benefit from the improved morale that can be evoked in the mothers by expanding their range of social experiences through the world of work. However, such assistance should be offered as an expression of society's positive concern and appreciation of the major responsibility of the women in rearing their children under very impoverished conditions. A punitive approach can never be effective and is incompatible with President Clinton's expression of compassion for the poor.

In research interviews, these mothers have shown their determination to keep their children out of foster care. Their labors are necessary to prevent the criminalization of their children. There should be careful effort not to disrupt parental functioning as we move toward reform of income maintenance. Not only do the families require adequate day care, but careful assessments are required concerning the effects of new program demands upon parental performance of the young women.

YOUNG PARENTS: KEY PLAYERS IN THE WAR AGAINST CRIME

In the course of their daily work, social workers bear witness to the suffering of children living in the midst of extreme poverty and social disorganization. They see parents struggling to carry out their responsibilities under very stressful conditions. Typically, income insufficiency and the lack of decent housing are exacerbated by the presence of criminal activities and rampant drug use in the communities in which the families reside. The ability of the parents to resist the noxious influences at play is highly dependent upon the provision of services supported by federal and state programs. Our focus is upon social policies reflected in legislation and administrative regulations that determine the adequacy of funding and the mandates under which service programs operate.

Stressed-out parents who are slacking in their parental functioning, because of the mean nature of their living circumstances, are prone to serious neglect and abuse of their children. Such children become candidates for delinquent behaviors in childhood followed by criminal careers in adulthood. In a follow-up study of former foster children in the state of Washington, my colleagues and I found that the physical abuse of boys early in their lives was a significant predictor of antisocial life-course development extending into the adult years when involvement in serious crime took place.

Once a woman gives birth to a child, even under circumstances that are not in her own or the child's interests, the community has a stake in her well-being and adequate functioning as a parent. Parent and child must be able to bond together in a loving relationship. This has long been our national goal in Republican, as well as Democratic, administrations. The child's whole future is conditioned by the mother being able to assume maternal responsibilities in round-the-clock child care. While single-parent families are more prone to becoming marginal, it is striking that the majority of these young women rise to their responsibilities and are able to provide security for their children.

These women are impoverished, very much on their own as single mothers, and handicapped in the performance of parental tasks. While such a set of circumstances can clearly have serious negative consequences for the child who is the product of such a union, it does not follow that the mother has less value for the child than is true of other youngsters born under more favorable circumstances. On the contrary, the child living under marginal economic and social circumstances is likely to exhibit an exceptionally high degree of emotional dependency. The anxious clinging of such children to their mothers is frequently observed by pediatricians, teachers, social workers, and public health nurses in the course of professional contacts with such families.

CHILD WELFARE IMPLICATIONS
OF THE TRANSFORMATION OF THE WELFARE SYSTEM

"You let loose a lot of forces when you say, 'End welfare as we know it,' which is why I never said any such thing," said

Senator Daniel Patrick Moynihan last spring, as the proposals raced to the right. "We may look back and say, 'What in name of God have we done?'" (Quoted by Jason DeParle, *The New York Times,* December 18, 1994)

The forces have been let loose. The Clinton administration has already given waivers to four states that allow them to deny additional benefits for a child born to a family already receiving AFDC. Other states are following suit with a plethora of new regulations. The changes being implemented by the states and contemplated in the Republican Contract with America, under the Personal Responsibility Act, are momentous.

It is prudent at this juncture to bear in mind that a vast literature on social program evaluations suggests that well-intentioned changes of this kind are difficult to execute without many families and children falling between the cracks.

The child welfare systems across the country, comprised of public and private agencies, will be called upon within the next few years to repair the damage. These systems are not prepared for the massive rise in caseloads that the United States surely will face.

It has been known since 1991 that child welfare services are in disarray. A bipartisan National Commission on Children established by the United States Congress issued a major report assessing the status of the country's children and the service system designed to minister to their needs. The Commission was dismayed by what it had learned.

> If the nation had deliberately designed a system that would frustrate the professionals who staff it, anger the public who finance it, and abandon the children who depend on it, it could not have done a better job than the present child welfare system. . . . The National Commission on Children heard from virtually every actor in the system: child welfare staff and dependency court judges who want more manageable caseloads so they can give children and families the thoughtful attention they need; foster parents who need more training and support to meet the developmental needs of children who arrive at their homes with chronic illnesses, disabilities, and severe emotional problems; families who wish someone had

reached out to them earlier; and foster children who want what all children want—a loving, safe, and nurturing family and a stable, secure home. Marginal changes will not turn this system around. Instead we need comprehensive reform based on fundamental restructuring of our efforts to help troubled children and protect vulnerable children.[8]

ACCOUNTABILITY: A MORAL IMPERATIVE

It is a moral imperative that a formal accounting be carried out about the consequences of welfare reform. In evaluative studies, it is essential that status outcomes related to the child's survivorship and care arrangements include counts of infanticide, abandonment of infants (in dumpsters and other places), surrendering of infants for adoption, and placement of children in foster care. It is also required that information be gathered about the condition of the children with respect to developmental progress and their overall physical and mental well-being. Given the seriousness of the issues, a major investment in longitudinal studies of large samples of the children using enriched descriptive data bases is necessary. There is no indication in current federal budgetary planning that investigations of this kind will be supported.

UNINTENDED CONSEQUENCES OF SOCIAL POLICY CHANGES

It is hoped by those promoting the new welfare rules that the effect of the withdrawal of public welfare support will be that teenagers will be encouraged to move toward abstinence from sexual relations and thus not embark upon premature parental careers. The literature does not support optimism about changing adolescent sexual behavior although some programs are reporting success using less coercive methods. The major psychological impact of the withholding of support is likely to come *after* the teenager discovers she is pregnant.

PREDICTING A MAJOR RISE
IN YOUNG WOMEN SEEKING ABORTIONS

The subject that has been studiously avoided in the debates on welfare reform is the probability of a sharp rise in the number of women seeking abortions. Under the new policies, the expectant mother who is a teenager would be faced with the prospect of not being able to bond with her child in an independent domicile and/or without assured income support. She would have to contemplate traveling on a very difficult road as a parent. Under the conditions of reality shock, the most attractive escape from the situation for a large portion of the teenagers would be to secure an abortion.

The expectation of a major rise in teenage abortions in the coming period is influenced by the following facts. One million teenage women become pregnant each year. In 1992, there were 406,000 abortions obtained by teenagers.[9] Absent from their ranks were those who decided to go to full term in their pregnancies and obtained AFDC support. Further, it is known that about half of all unwed teen mothers go on welfare within one year of the birth of their child.[10]

A modest increase, say 10 percent, in abortions obtained by young women who would otherwise chose maternal careers with AFDC support has to be seen as a conservative estimate given the lack of options facing women under the new welfare arrangements. This amounts to about 40,000 cases if the overall abortion rate continues at the 1992 level.

It is possible that groups normally in opposition to each other in the abortion debate that has raged in the United States over several decades will share a common antipathy to legislation that stimulates a rise of historic proportions in the number of women seeking abortion. A most eloquent argument against the Republican-sponsored legislation has already been made by the National Conference of Catholic Bishops. The Conference's president Archbishop William H. Keeler of Baltimore is reported in a *New York Times* editorial (November 24, 1994) as having warned against "punitive welfare provisions" that would destroy fragile families and bury children deeper in poverty. Archbishop Keeler said the bishops' opposition to such cruelty was not partisan, but based on the Church's teachings about the dignity of life.

Can right-to-life and pro-choice groups join forces to oppose the explosion in abortions that will result from severe policies directed at the poor? One can dream the impossible dream.

INVITING A SOCIAL DISASTER

The tragic and momentous events leading to large-scale rioting and fire setting in Los Angeles in May 1992 brought to the fore demands that our domestic agenda be addressed. The plight of poor families in the inner cities clearly helped create a powder keg that can explode unpredictably. This was recognized by both President Bush and President Clinton.

This sense of potential explosiveness of inept policymaking is revealed in the following excerpt reported by DeParle in his powerful description of the struggle of a woman to avoid depending upon welfare assistance in *The New York Times Magazine* on December 18, 1994:

> The sudden popularity of the literal end of welfare took even a credentialed conservative like [Representative Rick] Santorum by surprise. "The risk is that you are going to have millions of women and children with absolutely no support out there," he said last spring. Moynihan tartly predicted "scenes of social trauma such as we haven't known since the cholera epidemic."

FROM POVERTY TO MISERY

While in exile in the United States, the President of Haiti, Jean-Bertrand Aristide, described his economic aspirations for the desperately impoverished people of Haiti as that of raising them from "misery to poverty." The data on inequality of income in the United States, the information we have on the severe erosion that has taken place in the level of income assistance to families receiving public assistance, and the threats to cut many families off welfare assistance entirely indicates that we are moving in the direction of lowering the economic status of the poor in the United States from "poverty to misery."

NOTES

1. Polsky, H. (1962). *Cottage six*. New York: Russell Sage Foundation.

2. Herstein, N. (1965). A critique of current research in child welfare. In *The known and the unknown in child welfare research*. New York: Child Welfare League of America and National Association of Social Workers (Joint publication), pp. 82-104.

3. Wulczyn, F. H. (1992). *Status at birth and infant foster care placement in New York City*. Albany: New York State Department of Social Services.

4. Fanshel, D., Finch, S. J., and Grundy, J. F. (1992). *Serving the urban poor*. Westport, CN: Praeger.

5. National Center for Children in Poverty. *Young children in poverty: A statistical update*. New York: Columbia University School of Public Health, 1994.

6. Pear, R. "G.O.P. affirms plan to stop money for unwed mothers." *The New York Times*, January 21, 1995.

7. Ibid.

8. National Commission on Children. (1991). Beyond rhetoric: A new American agenda for children and families. Final Report. Washington, DC: National Commission on Children, p. 293.

9. The Alan Guttmacher Institute. *Facts in brief: Abortion in the United States*. New York: Author. August 31, 1994.

10. Besharov, D. J. The other Clinton promise—Ending "welfare as we know it." *The Wall Street Journal*, January 13, 1993.

Chapter 4

Mandatory versus Voluntary HIV Testing of Newborns

Nilsa S. Gutierrez

One of the most controversial health policy questions in the last two years and, in fact, in the history of the HIV (human immuno-deficiency virus) epidemic in New York State, is HIV testing of newborns. This issue has challenged fundamental principles of HIV care, principles that have been delineated through long and painful experience with this devastating disease and have been conserved as the supporting structure for all of New York's HIV prevention and treatment programs. Public discussion has polarized opinion rather than encouraged consensus. The issue has once again brought the political context of HIV/AIDS prevention and care into sharp relief.

What is the issue and why is it so provocative? The tragedy of HIV infection in children prompts all health care professionals and planners to seek ways to prevent HIV transmission from mothers to infants and to more efficiently identify infected children and bring them into treatment. Mandatory HIV testing of all newborns has been proposed as one way to identify infected infants.

There are a number of reasons why nearly all major health profes-sional organizations oppose mandatory newborn testing and instead support mandatory prenatal HIV counseling, together with medically recommended voluntary HIV testing, for women in all health settings.

Mandatory newborn testing does not accurately identify infected infants at birth, does not ensure access to treatment, violates New York State law requiring informed consent by testing mothers invol-untarily, and, perhaps most importantly, is too late to reduce the risk of HIV transmission to infants.

In contrast, prenatal identification of women with HIV infection allows earlier detection of infants exposed to HIV; establishes a cooperative relationship between women and health care providers, which leads to improved medical care for women and children; and gives pregnant women options that may prevent the transmission of HIV to their infants. Some background may help explain these points.

First, although mandatory newborn testing seems to be a quick and accurate way to find all HIV-infected newborns, it is, in fact, neither quick nor error-free. The HIV test in current use does not identify the presence of the virus itself, but tests for antibodies to the virus in the blood. A positive HIV test in an adult indicates a definite HIV infection. However, while every baby born to a woman with HIV will test positive, only 20 to 25 percent of infants are actually infected. The others are carrying HIV antibodies from the mother, which disappear within a few months.

There is currently no test that can tell at birth which babies are definitely infected although the polymerase chain reaction (PCR) test can make this distinction at about one month of age. PCR is expensive and is not used as an initial screening tool, but is available as of April 1995 free of charge to every infant born to a women with known HIV infection. It is expected that infants exposed to HIV in utero will require several PCR tests beginning about a month after birth to determine their true HIV status.

Although an antibody test does not reveal which newborns are infected, it does indicate which mothers are infected. That is why mandatory testing of newborns is actually mandatory testing of mothers. Current New York State law does not allow mandatory HIV testing of any population although federal law requires HIV testing of all federal prisoners, applicants for permanent residency, and Job Corps applicants.

Currently AIDS cases, that is, people with HIV infection who meet the definition of AIDS determined by the federal Centers for Disease Control and Prevention (CDC), are reported to health officials, but other cases of HIV infection are not reported. Therefore, there is no accurate way to measure the rate of HIV infection in any group.

However, the number of newborns with maternal antibodies does provide a measure of the rate of HIV infection in women who give birth in any one year. The CDC conducts a study in 45 states, the HIV Survey in Childbearing Women, which is an anonymous survey of the rate of maternal HIV infection as revealed by tests for HIV antibodies in newborns. New York State has participated in the survey since 1987, testing the blood of nearly every newborn in New York State for HIV and using the results to plan HIV prevention, testing, and treatment services for women and children.

In this study, in accordance with the national study design and New York State law, a portion of a blood sample from each newborn is sent for HIV testing with no identifying information about the mother or infant. Thus, the study is a "blinded" research tool, not a public-health screening program. It does not conform to any of the legal requirements for HIV testing programs, which include pre- and posttest counseling and informed consent.

In 1993, New York State Assemblywoman Nettie Mayersohn from Queens introduced a bill in the Assembly Health Committee that became known as the AIDS Baby Bill, a proposal to "unblind" the anonymous newborn seroprevalence survey. The intent was to require the state to inform mothers when an infant tested positive so that HIV-infected infants could receive care as soon as possible and infected mothers would avoid breastfeeding, another route of HIV transmission to infants.

The State Assembly asked the State's AIDS Advisory Council, which reports to the governor and oversees the work of the AIDS Institute, to establish a subcommittee to study the question.

The subcommittee did not support "unblinding" the study or mandatory newborn testing, calling instead for mandatory HIV counseling for women in all settings where women received health care. They urged that physicians strongly recommend HIV testing to any woman who was pregnant or thinking of pregnancy, but that the test itself remain voluntary. They further recommended that pediatricians who did not know a child's HIV status provide HIV counseling to the mother and strongly advise HIV testing.

Another bill was introduced by State Senator Michael Tully, Chair of the Senate Health Committee, which attempted to codify the policy of mandatory counseling. This bill was passed by the Senate. In the Assembly, a separate bill supporting mandatory counseling was introduced by Speaker Sheldon Silver and Health Committee Chair Richard Gottfried and was passed. However, thus far no bill has passed both houses of the legislature, and the governor has now asked his Task Force on Life and the Law to consider the issue. Legislators have every expectation that bills on newborn HIV screening will be reintroduced at the next session.

HIV PRINCIPLES OF CARE

Current public health law concerning HIV in New York and all HIV programs share some basic principles that have also shaped New York State policy on newborn testing.

First, state health officials believe that every person should know his or her HIV status. The Department of Health has always maintained the importance of HIV counseling and testing to prevent the spread of HIV to sexual partners. Although initially the test was recommended only to people thought to be high risk, now all adults and adolescents who are or have been sexually active are encouraged to learn their HIV status. Informed consent is required in all testing programs as proof that clients understand what the test is for.

Pre- and posttest counseling has long been an essential part of HIV education in New York to teach people to protect themselves and their partners and to ensure that those who test positive receive treatment.

Voluntarism and confidentiality are the other cornerstones of New York State HIV/AIDS policy. Throughout the epidemic, despite repeated calls for mandatory HIV testing of various populations, New York has been firm in its commitment to education and voluntary testing as the most effective way to bring people with HIV infection into care. Confidentiality is critical to the success of counseling and testing programs since many people would be reluctant to come for testing if the government, their employers, their landlords, or anyone else had access to information about their HIV status.

In fact, the earliest statewide HIV counseling and testing programs, established by the AIDS Institute immediately after the development of the HIV antibody test in 1985, were anonymous. At anonymous sites, no one knows the identity of the person being tested and clients use a number rather than a name to sign the consent form.

The New York City Health Department currently runs nine such programs, and 43 others are run by State Health Department.

At all other settings, HIV testing is confidential. The client's name is linked to the test sample and the results are recorded in the medical record. Access to information about the client and the test result is strictly controlled at the testing site, but breaches of confidentiality do happen occasionally.

In 1989, New York State Public Health Law Article 27-F standardized the pre- and posttest counseling process and gave the principles of voluntarism, confidentiality, and informed consent the weight of law.

These policies have been reviewed several times specifically in relation to women. The Mohonk Principles, named for the conference sponsored by the Department of Health at the Mohonk Mountain House in January of 1990, and the report of the second Mohonk conference in January 1992 continued to support anonymous and confidential testing rather than mandatory testing. The report suggested offering HIV counseling as a routine part of care for all women of reproductive age.

The opposition to unblinding the HIV Survey of Childbearing Women and to newborn mandatory testing in general is a reconfirmation of the soundness of these principles.

Mandatory testing of newborns, which is involuntary testing of mothers, challenges the requirement that every person give informed consent for an HIV test. It does not provide for counseling or treatment of mothers or children, and it is not strictly confidential if a woman's husband, partner, or other family members can learn her status through the baby's test result.

Besides the fact that any mandatory newborn testing program could violate state law in these ways and that unblinding the current anonymous program would violate the requirements of the national HIV Survey of Childbearing Women, there are practical and medical reasons for opposition to mandatory newborn testing.

While all medical care is dependent on cooperative relationships with health care providers, HIV care for infants is directly dependent on the voluntary cooperation and active participation of mothers or, in some cases, guardians. Infants exposed to HIV must be brought in for PCR testing at about one month of age to confirm the

HIV diagnosis and, if infected, to begin treatment. Most mothers want what is best for their children and will bring children for medical care, but this is most likely when mothers have trusting relationships with health care providers and when counseling and testing is not coercive or required.

There is perhaps an even more critical reason to focus on prenatal HIV counseling and testing of mothers rather than HIV testing of newborns. Identification of HIV-infected women during pregnancy gives health care providers the chance to help women prevent HIV transmission to their infants. This is a very compelling reason for a woman to agree to HIV testing, even if she is not concerned about her own status.

HIV infection can be passed from mother to child at any point in the birth process: during pregnancy, during delivery, or after delivery through breastfeeding. Dramatic preliminary results from a federal study known as AIDS Clinical Trial Group 076 showed a two-thirds reduction in risk of HIV for infants born to mothers who had taken zidovudine (AZT) during pregnancy. Only 8 percent of these infants were HIV infected, compared to 25 percent of the control group.

Physicians who counsel and identify infected women during pregnancy have the opportunity to discuss the use of ZDV and the need to test infants a month after birth. They can also advise women with HIV infection prior to childbirth to avoid breastfeeding. Counseling to prevent breastfeeding by HIV-infected mothers has been a long-standing recommendation of the Department of Health.

Newborn HIV testing would do nothing to reduce the risk of HIV transmission to infants during or even after pregnancy. Currently, it takes nearly one month to receive results of standard HIV antibody tests although with additional staff and funding, the results could be available in five days. Still, in five days most mothers have already left the hospital and have begun breastfeeding. Confirmation of the HIV diagnosis using PCR takes at least one month.

Some who support mandatory newborn testing have wanted to add HIV to the list of seven congenital diseases for which the state currently screens all newborns. However, HIV is not like these other diseases or the two (syphilis and hepatitis B) for which New York screens pregnant women. All of these diseases are treatable and do not imply an inevitably fatal illness for the mother or child. Further, by law, parents must be told of the reasons for congenital disease testing, and they can refuse testing on religious grounds. Test results are not provided to parents, but to health care providers who must find and notify parents, which is often a difficult task.

The State Department of Health position on newborn screening is consistent with the view that informs all of its policies: HIV/AIDS is different from other diseases and requires unique types of programs and solutions.

HIV AND AIDS
IN NEW YORK WOMEN AND CHILDREN

Some figures may help to put the problem into perspective. From 1981, at the start of data collection, through June 30, 1994, nearly 20 percent of New York's more than 77,000 cumulative cases of AIDS were women. About two-thirds of people diagnosed with AIDS have died. Just over 52 percent of New York women with AIDS since 1981 have been black; 31 percent have been Hispanic, and 16 percent have been white.

Looking at the increase in women's cases by year gives a more accurate assessment. In 1993, 25 percent of new AIDS cases were in women, a percentage that has increased steadily each year from 16 percent in 1988.

Of infected women, about 60 percent are active or former drug users. Heterosexual transmission, accounting for about 30 percent of AIDS cases in women, is rapidly on the rise and is a much higher risk for women than for men. A fair amount of the heterosexual transmission to women is also from drug-using partners.

There have been 1,500 cases of AIDS in children under age 13 since 1981, with approximately the same racial distribution as AIDS in women. In 1993, there were 148 new cases of AIDS in children under 13 years of age.

AIDS cases in adults are an indication of HIV infection rates five to eight years prior to AIDS diagnosis, the average time to progress from HIV infection to a CDC-defined case of AIDS. Estimating total current HIV infection in New York State is still difficult.

Although there is no estimate of the HIV infection rate among all women of childbearing age, the HIV Survey of Childbearing Women reports that among the 300,000 women who give birth in one year in New York State the HIV-infection rate has decreased from .66 percent in 1989 to .57 percent in 1993.

In 1993, 1,576 HIV-infected women gave birth. Nearly 90 percent of these women were black or Hispanic. About 25 percent of New York hospitals account for nearly 90 percent of births to infected women, which take place for the most part in New York City.

Since 20 to 25 percent of the infants born to women with HIV will actually be infected, in 1993, that would be 314 to 394 new cases of HIV in newborns.

About half of women with infected infants know their HIV status at the time of delivery through the programs funded by the AIDS Institute. An undetermined additional number know their status through non–state-funded programs or private physicians.

VOLUNTARY HIV COUNSELING AND TESTING

There is a wide range of counseling and testing programs in New York State to encourage women to be tested for HIV at any point before, during, or after childbirth. The recommendation is that every pregnant woman or every woman considering pregnancy learn her current HIV status, even if she has been tested before.

In one 1990 national survey, more than two-thirds of voluntary HIV tests were obtained in private settings, such as physicians' offices and HMOs. Besides these, HIV test settings in New York State include all of the facilities funded specifically to do HIV counseling and testing. These include the Designated AIDS Centers and Maternal/Pediatrics programs in hospitals; the family planning, substance abuse, and sexually transmitted disease clinics; community health centers; the Prenatal Care Assistance Program; prisons; anonymous test sites; and the Obstetrical Initiative, which counsels and tests women at the time of childbirth.

The performance of the "voluntary testing program" has been compared to a hypothetical "mandatory testing" program. In fact, there are many types of voluntary programs. Each of the HIV test settings has its own very particular environment and its own fairly consistent level of performance. Data by type of site range from 20 or 30 percent test acceptance to more than 90 percent.

HIV testing is never an end in itself. It must be part of a continuum of care that stretches from community education to terminal illness. The AIDS Institute has always insisted that testing be closely linked to prevention and treatment services and that hospitals work with community providers in referral networks.

Many different types of people are responsible for HIV counseling. The counselor may be a physician, nurse, physician's assistant, social worker, health technician, community health worker, homeless shelter worker, student, or volunteer. Counseling may be done by all staff members at a facility or it may be the exclusive job of a specially designated HIV counselor.

Despite long-standing efforts to standardize the counseling process, what clients actually experience varies considerably with the type of setting, the specific facility, and the individual counselor. Nonphysician counselors in state-funded programs complete a program of counselor training. Although counseling programs undergo regular evaluation, there are insufficient resources to determine how individual counselors perform or whether all follow the state-mandated counseling format.

Many factors influence counseling effectiveness, including knowledge and attitude of the counselor; administrative and institutional support; integration of HIV counseling and testing with routine health care; availability of basic support services such as adequate staff and blood-drawing facilities; convenient hours; cultural similarities between counselor and client; frequency of client exposure to HIV information; and a client's sense of individual risk.

Further, a diagnosis of HIV infection provokes many social problems. A woman may not be willing to inform her spouse or partner of a positive test for fear of violence or other abuse. A monogamous woman may not be willing to accuse her partner of infidelity. Besides HIV monitoring and medical care, affected families may need help with substance abuse treatment, insurance, child-care, custody arrangements, wills, transportation, nutrition, and often housing.

The AIDS Institute has continually reviewed the ability of its voluntary programs to reach women, persuade them to be tested, and provide treatment and support services. While different programs function very differently, in general over the past three years programs have shown the following: (1) a decrease in the rate of HIV infection among clients; (2) an increase in the rate at which clients return for test results; and (3) fairly consistent variation among the rates of test acceptance in different test settings.

Counseling and testing rates above 80 percent are generally achieved in sites that have highly motivated, well-coordinated, inter-disciplinary staff, such as in some hospitals, substance abuse treatment programs, and community health centers. Where women get intermittent care, when there is no relationship between the woman and the health care provider, or when the provider is not the woman's primary care physician, test acceptance is lower.

The Obstetrical Initiative is a program that has been attacked for low test-acceptance rates. It was not designed as a principal HIV testing program but as a fail-safe effort to counsel women in obstetrical settings who had not been counseled or tested for HIV before. These were often women who had not received any prenatal care and were at very high risk for HIV, although the program found that a large number of women who had had prenatal care had never been offered HIV counseling.

The program provides HIV counseling and testing immediately after childbirth, which is a very difficult time. An internal study of the Obstetrical Initiative in 1992 indicated that the best predictors for test acceptance were the length of time the counselor spent with the client and the identity of the counselor. Some counselors in one hospital had a 3 percent test acceptance rate and others in the same hospital achieved 90 percent. More than 45 minutes with a female counselor resulted in a test-acceptance rate of 77 percent. Less than 15 minutes produced only a 16 percent acceptance rate. Some counselors had misconceptions about the epidemic, about HIV, transmission, treatment, and services.

In research on family planning programs and the Prenatal Care Assistance Program by Columbia University's School of Public Health, women said they declined an HIV test because they already knew their HIV status, they did not want to know, or they thought they had not been exposed to HIV.

Women often did not recall counseling information. Some did not believe that the HIV test identified the virus for AIDS. Some thought that physicians should know a client's status, but the client should not. Some believed they must have been tested already without their consent. There was misunderstanding about transmission of HIV and belief that there are no treatment options. Some, especially African-American women, thought the HIV epidemic was a genocidal plan.

CURRENT HIV POLICY

The misinformation, despite more than ten years of public education, lends support to the prediction that some women will avoid the health care system completely if mandatory HIV testing were imposed. A reduction in prenatal care or regular health care or an unwillingness to come to the hospital to give birth would have serious negative consequences for infants at risk for HIV.

Some wonder whether the state could force women to bring their HIV-positive children for treatment, even before the diagnosis was confirmed, and make it a criminal activity to refuse such treatment based on fear of or uncertainty about new drugs. Others worry about losing custody of their children, homelessness, or other repercussions of learning their HIV status.

The Department of Health, through the AIDS Institute, has worked with community groups to clarify policy and information about HIV treatment. It has also worked to improve the uneven performance of counseling and testing programs and has allocated an additional $6 million to expand statewide HIV services for women and children.

Current New York State Department of Health policy recommends routine, universal HIV counseling, and medically recommended voluntary HIV testing for every woman in every health care setting. The AIDS Institute and major medical and public health professional organizations remain opposed to mandatory testing and convinced that the best care for children will come from voluntary prenatal counseling and testing of mothers.

Chapter 5

The Changing Structure of African-American Families

Andrew Billingsley

The family continues to be the most important and most highly valued aspect of African-American life. As late as 1990, for example, some 70 percent of all African-American households were family households. This means that according to the U.S. Census, these households were occupied by two or more persons related to each other by marriage, lineage, or adoption. Still another measure of the salience of the family among African-American people is that the majority of black men over age 30 are currently married and living with their spouse. Still another is that whenever young black people under age 20 are asked whether they plan to be married, a majority answer in the affirmative. Yet another fact: Of the more than one million black children unable to live with their natural parents, for a variety of reasons, the overwhelming majority—up to 80 percent—of them are being raised by relatives, not the foster care system. Or consider the following: A majority of black adults are not poor (only about one-third are poor), and among the nonpoor black adults, a majority live in two-parent family households. The same may be said of unemployment. A majority of black adults are employed, and among the employed, a majority live in two-parent family households. Let me present one final statistic. There are currently more black families in existence than ever before. The total number of black families in the nation rose from 6.5 million in 1983 to more than 7.2 million by 1990, which is an increase over the year before. Moreover, the number of black married couples has also continued to increase. In 1983, there were some 3.5 million black married couples in the nation. By 1990, this number had increased to 3.8 million, up from 3.7 million the year before. Finally, married couples come in two types. Married couples with children and married couples without children. By 1990 among the 3.8 million black two-parent families, a slight majority were married with children of their own under age 18. Altogether, 2.0 million had young children of their own while 1.8 million black married couples were without children of their own living with them.

These numbers add up to the fact that the family is a large and growing presence among the more than 30 million African-American people, even at the present time.

This is far from the prevailing portrait of African-American families in public discourse. How do we get a correct and perceptive picture of African-American family life today? The approach advocated is to take a broad, holistic perspective toward this phenomenon taking into consideration the historical evolution of family life in black America and the broad societal context within which family life occurs. In *Black Families in White America*, I referred to this as a Social Systems Approach to the study of black family life. Propositions which should guide the study of these families are as follows:

1. The whole is greater than its parts.
2. History is prologue.
3. Society has the upper hand in the shaping of families.
4. Family structure is adaptive.
5. The African-American community is generative.
6. The future is already here.

I explore each proposition in *Climbing Jacob's Ladder: The Enduring Legacy of African-American Families*. This chapter will focus, however, on the changing structure of African-American families although several of these other propositions will also be discussed.

FAMILY STRUCTURAL DIVERSITY

The search for the meaning of recent transformation in the African-American community must take into consideration that no single family form characterizes the black community. Instead, a wide variety of structures have arisen. For the 100-year period between the end of slavery and the aftermath of World War II, the structure of African-American family life was characterized by a remarkable degree of stability. Three structures characterize this traditional African-American family system. Specifically, the core of the traditional African-American family system has been the nuclear family composed of husband and wife and their own children. A second element in the traditional African-American family system is the extended family, a carryover from African heritage. Often, the nuclear core was augmented by other relatives, creating the extended family. A third element in this family tradition is the augmented family form. Sometimes the nuclear core and extended relatives were joined by nonrelatives, creating the augmented family. This, then, is the traditional African-American family system. It is not the same as the traditional American family system. Most black adults today are familiar with this traditional family system: The system consists of the nuclear core, surrounded by extended relatives, and often augmented by nonrelatives as well. The stability of this family system is reflected by the fact that during the years between slavery and the 1960s, a majority of African-American families had married couples at their core, and a majority of children were reared by two parents plus other relatives. Indeed, it has been pointed out that the net decline in black married-couple families between 1890 and 1960 was less than 10 percent through the entire period. Among all black men, the proportion married declined from 67 percent in 1890 to 64 percent in 1960. Among women, it ranged from 56 percent to 58 percent over this period. After the 1960s, however, the decline became phenomenal, and the traditional African-American family structure began to give way to a wide variety of alternative forms.

As late as 1960, when uneducated black men could still hold good-paying blue-collar jobs in the industrial sector, fully 78 percent of all black families with children were headed by married couples. By 1970, only 64 percent of African-American families with children were headed by married couples. This declined steadily to 54 percent by 1975, to 48 percent by 1980, and to a minority of 40 percent by 1985. This trend is likely to continue in the future. Meanwhile, one of the alternatives to the traditional family, the single-parent family—particularly the female-headed family—has escalated enormously over the past generation. Consisting of a minority of 22 percent of families with children in 1960, this family form had increased to 33 percent by 1970, to 49 percent by 1980, and to a whopping 57 percent by 1985.

Thus, beginning in 1980 for the first time in history, female-headed families with children outnumbered married-couple families with children. It also means that for the first time since slavery, a majority of black children lived in single-parent families. This, too, will continue to increase in the future. While black married-couple families are projected to increase by 11 percent between now and the year 2000, the number of female-headed families will increase by 25 percent. Thus, the nuclear, extended, and augmented family forms, which were adopted after slavery and which were to serve the African-American people well for 125 years, are all in a rapid state of decline.

The decline in the marriage relation, which stands at the center of the African-American family crisis, has been so sharp and sustained in recent years that a number of observers have begun to talk of the "vanishing black family." Indeed, a national forum at University of California, Los Angeles in 1989 brought together a group of leading black and white students of the black family to examine the future of marriage among African Americans.

The abandonment of the marriage relation is severe among both black males and females. The decline has been greater, however, among females. Thus, among adult black males, 18 and over, the proportion married declined dramatically from an overwhelming majority of 67 percent in 1970 to a bare majority of 51 percent by 1985. Meanwhile, the proportion of black women who were married plunged from a similar majority of 63 percent in 1970 to a minority of 43 percent by 1985.

These trends do not support the commonly held view that black men have a weaker attachment or commitment to marriage than black women. Indeed, it may suggest just the opposite. The fact that the proportion married is higher, the proportion divorced is lower, and the proportion remarried is also higher among men may suggest that black men have a greater attachment to marriage. Nonetheless, the observation here is that both black men and women have been avoiding or abandoning the marital status in record numbers during recent years. This behavior constitutes the leading edge of the contemporary African-American family crisis, but this is more a crisis in the marriage relation than in the family. Marriage, as I have pointed out, is one of several bases for family formation and endurance.

What, then, has taken the place of the traditional family system? At least six alternative family structures have arisen in postindustrial America to characterize the contemporary pattern of African-American family diversity.

Single-Person Households

First, increasing numbers of African-American adults are living in single-person households. They are single either because they have never married or have been married and separated, widowed, or divorced. Young persons are delaying marriage longer than in former years. Many are deciding to forego marriage altogether. The norms of society no longer require that persons be married in order to live respectable, healthy, and happy lives.

The world of single black adults has expanded enormously in recent years. As late as 1975, only 11 percent of black men, ages 35 to 44, were still single. These figures had not changed appreciably since 1890. The proportion of single black women was slightly lower and also steady at about 8 percent over this period.

After 1980, however, the population of single black adults rose dramatically. Not only were large numbers remaining unmarried, but also substantial proportions of those were choosing to live apart from their families in single-person households.

In 1983, of the 8.9 million black households in the nation, a total of 2.056 million were single-person households, with adults living alone. This represented 23 percent of all black households. Women outnumbered men slightly at 1.12 million to 934,000.

By 1986, these numbers had increased to 2.5 million, constituting 26 percent of the 9.8 million black households in that year. Single females living alone continued to outnumber single men.

This does not mean, of course, that they are absent family relationships. As we have observed above, they may have quite strong family ties, relationships, and responsibilities without living in the same household.

Cohabitation

A second alternative to the traditional family is cohabitation. Small but expanding numbers of adults are choosing to live with another person of the opposite sex and sometimes of the same sex in a marriage-like relationship without benefit of legal marriage. While fewer than 5 percent of black adults live in cohabitation relationships, this number is also expanding rapidly. Some do so as a prelude to marriage. Others do so in the aftermath of marriage. Still others pursue cohabitation as an alternative to marriage. Social norms have changed so drastically in recent years that, even in the black community, cohabitation—which has a long history, referred to as "shacking up"—has come to be quite acceptable and almost respectable. These arrangements tend, however, to be short lived and less stable than conventional marriages.

The number of cohabitating couples is difficult to know. In addition to the unmarried persons living in single-person households, large numbers live to two-person households with persons to whom they are not married and not related. In 1983, there were 266,000 such couples representing 2.9 percent of all black households. By 1986, these numbers had increased to 297,000, accounting for 3.2 percent of all living arrangements. This is the most likely pool from where cohabitating couples may be found.

Children, No Marriage

Among the most rapidly expanding family structures are those in which there are children without marriage. In 1983, there were 3.043 million black single-parent households (as compared with 3.486 million married-couple households and 2.386 million nonfamily households). Of these, 1.989 million were single parents with children under age eighteen. Of these, 127,000 were male-headed families and 1.864 million were female-headed families. Even this particular structure contains diversity. The 872,000 female-headed black families, all of whose children are age eighteen and over, must surely be distinguished from the 1.8 million who have children under age eighteen.

What is the source of their single-parent status? Among men 98,000 were never married, 79,000 were divorced, 68,000 were widowed, and 64,000 were married with absent spouses due to separation, incarceration, long-term illness, or desertion.

Among women, the same pattern existed. The largest percentage of these women were never married, comprising 899,000. Next, there were 655,000 divorced mothers, followed by 646,000 married with absent spouses and 534,000 widows with children.

By 1986, single-parent families from all sources had expanded. Overall, the number had increased to 3.242 million, representing 33 percent of the 9.8 million black households.

Married, No Children

A further deviation from traditional families is married couples without children. This type of family has also been expanding among African-American families. In 1983, there were 1.585 million black married couples without children. This represented 18 percent of all 8.9 million black households. By 1986, this had increased to 1.683 million, representing a similar proportion of the 9.8 million households.

Who are these couples without children? They are generally the more highly educated, higher income, two-earner families.

Not only is this an expanding family form, but it is also a highly satisfactory one. Our studies show that married partners without children exhibit the highest level of personal satisfaction, family satisfaction, and satisfaction with life in general, with higher self-esteem than that found in persons in any other type of family structure.

Married with Children

Finally, we come to a family pattern that approaches the traditional. These are married couples with children. In 1983, there were 1.901 million of these families, exceeding slightly the number of couples without children. Altogether, they accounted for 21 percent of the 8.9 million black households.

By 1986, despite population growth, there were still only 1.997 million black married-couple families with children. This amounted to a declining 20 percent of the 9.8 million black households.

Children and Relatives

Parents are not the only persons to head families. Grandparents still play an important role in extended families. Altogether there were 548,000 black extended families in 1983, accounting for 6 percent of the 8.9 million households. By 1986, this had expanded to 607,000 extended families, representing a similar proportion of the 9.8 million households.

By 1986, the mix had changed somewhat, with a substantial increase in the number of single-parent families taking in other relatives and a slight decline in the number of married couples doing so.

Still another arrangement increasingly common in the black community is a type of extended family in which children live with relatives, usually grandparents, quite apart from their parents altogether.

All these diverse family structures, now common and growing, constitute the essence of contemporary African-American family life. Some are involuntary; some are temporary and transitional. Some are filled with pain and suffering. All, however, have arisen to fill some need and function.

It is clear, moreover, that neither of the types of structures that have evolved is exclusive to African-American people. Because these types are driven by larger forces that affect the entire population, they appear in other groups as well. If the pattern is somewhat different among African Americans than among other American families, it is because of the realities of the African-American experience, which is also distinctive.

The key to understanding African-American family structure is to see the whole picture with its many variations and to note its flexibility. Almost no one remains throughout life in any one of these structures. Most adults pass through several family structures in the course of their lives. All single adults do not remain single. All cohabiting couples do not stay together permanently. All single mothers do not stay single, all married couples do not stay married, and all divorced persons do not remain divorced.

These structures represent, in part, the fallout from the decimation of the traditional family forms. They also represent, however, the remarkable capacity of these people to hold onto the spirit and the experience of family even in the face of this vanishing tradition.

Such flexibility, adaptability, and diversity are among the often underappreciated strengths of African-American families. This is why, on any given day, better than two-thirds of all African-American people will be found living in families of one form or another in the same proportion as in the nation at large. Many of those who live in single-person, or nonfamily households have substantial family relationships in actuality. All this suggests, as Mark Twain might have said, that the death of the African-American family has been greatly exaggerated.

SOCIAL-CLASS DIVERSITY

If the African-American people are characterized by diverse and rapidly changing patterns of family structure—rather than by any one family structure—this diversity is equally true with respect to social class. As important and troubling as is the celebrated "underclass," it represents only a small fraction of all African-American families who range across the entire spectrum of social classes. There are a number of reasons why it is important to take a holistic view of the African-American social class structure.

First, it helps to avoid stereotypes. A focus on only one stratum tends to suggest that it is characteristic of black families. Second, a view of the entire class structure helps to show that there is upward and downward mobility in operation. It shows, for example, that one class may be expanding at the expense of another or that one class may be the source of expansion in other classes. Additionally, a view of the entire class structure shows the dynamism in the African-American community. It helps to avoid the often-repeated suggestion that the underclass is permanent, or that there are only two classes—underclass and middle class, or that there is no black upper class, all of which are part of today's fashionable but false conventional wisdom.

More important, a view of the entire class spectrum will reveal that it is none of the mentioned classes but the black blue-collar working class that is the backbone of the black community. Finally, it will show that it is precisely this working class that is being decimated by changing technological, economic, and social conditions, which, in turn, constitute the major reason for the demise of traditional African-American family patterns. From the perspective of social change and reform, then, an appreciation of the entire social-class structure of the black community is important.

The concept social class suggests that some families have greater resources, higher status, and more options than others in managing their lives. The three most common indexes for measuring social class are the amount of family income, the educational level, and the occupational prestige of the head of the family. Each index has advantages and limitations. The family income measure is superior to the others as a measure of economic and social well-being.

Five Social Classes

In our own work, we have identified five distinct social class strata in the African-American community. Based primarily on level of family income, complemented by education, occupation, and style of life, these five strata include: (1) the underclass, consisting of poor families in which no member has a permanent attachment to the workforce; (2) the working poor, who, despite working for low wages, are not able to earn above the poverty line; (3) the nonpoor working class, composed of unskilled and semiskilled blue-collar workers with earnings above the poverty line; (4) the middle class, comprised primarily of white-collar skilled and professional workers with family income above the median for all families; and (5) a small black upper class of families with high incomes and substantial wealth as well as social and economic influence. Relying primarily on median combined family incomes converted into 1983 dollars, I have identified these five social-class strata at three points in time: 1969, 1983, and 1986.

One of the most striking features of the entire social-class structure is that while the underclass has been expanding over this period, the nonpoor working class was declining by almost the exact same magnitude, from 44 percent in 1969 to 36 percent in 1983 and to 34 percent of all African-American families by 1986. This shows with dramatic clarity that the underclass is expanding at the expense of the nonpoor working class. In turn, this removes a considerable amount of the mystery as to why the underclass is growing and from where this growth is coming.

The underclass, i.e., those families in which no member has a secure and productive niche in the workforce, is at the bottom of the social structure. These are overwhelmingly single-parent families with fully 75 percent single-parent and only 25 percent husband-wife families. Where did they come from? Some families in this stratum expanded by persons leaving one family and creating another underclass family without bettering their conditions. The birth of children to persons who moved out of their parents' home and formed new families is another. Just as surely, large numbers of these families were downwardly mobile from the working poor and the nonpoor working class. They became part of the underclass as the rapid march of technological change put millions of unskilled, uneducated, and inexperienced workers out of work.

Moving up the socioeconomic ladder, just above the underclass, we find a second stratum. These are families of the working poor. If we combine the nonworking poor with the working poor, we note that African-American families in poverty after declining dramatically in the 1960s expanded from 28 percent of the total in 1969 to 37 percent by 1983 before declining slightly to 30 percent by 1986. Consequently, poor black families nearly doubled, increasing from 1.4 million families in 1969 to more than 2.4 million by 1983. Even though the poverty rate had declined to 30 percent by 1986, there were still some 2.1 million poor black families in 1986—somewhat more than the 1.9 million in 1959 who constituted 46 percent of black families at that time. It is also important to note that poverty is not so permanent or intractable as some commentators suggest. Starting with a high of 46 percent of all black families in 1959, poverty was dramatically reduced to 26 percent by 1969 after a decade of reform. It remained steady through the 1970s and escalated sharply again during the 1980s. This analysis shows distinctly that some families are poor because they do not have work while others are poor despite having work at low-wage jobs in the labor force.

The working poor are those families in which at least one member is employed. They have median incomes below the poverty line due to low wages, including a minimum wage that has not kept pace with inflation. Even the rise in the minimum wage passed by Congress in 1988 is so far below inflation that it will lift few families out of poverty.

Only one-third of these working poor families are husband-wife families and as many have working husbands and wives. This stratum remained steady at 14 percent of all African-American families between 1969 and 1983. Because of the expanding population, the actual numbers of African-American families in the working poor stratum increased from 688,000 in 1969 to 963,000 by 1983. Thus, there were more working poor black families in 1983 than there had been in 1969.

If we combine the working nonpoor and the working poor, we note that the working class continues to comprise the largest sector of the African-American community, ranging downward from 58 percent of all African-American families in 1969 to 50 percent by 1983 and declining further by 1986. Where did they go? Some moved up to the expanding middle and upper classes. More, however, moved down to the expanding underclass.

Above the working poor in the socioeconomic structure is a sector we call the nonpoor working class. The nonpoor (or near poor) working class is composed of those families with combined family incomes ranging from just above the poverty line of $10,000 in 1983 dollars to just under $25,000. Composed largely of blue-collar, skilled, and unskilled workers, these families are less dependent on dual earners than the middle and upper classes. Only 45 percent have working wives and husbands. Most have a high school education.

This largely blue-collar nonpoor working class has declined dramatically since 1969. That year, some 44 percent of African-American families were in this class, comprising some 2.1 million families. This was and still is the largest single stratum serving as the economic, social, and political backbone of the black community. By 1983, this stratum had declined to 36 percent of all African-American families. Because of the expanding population, however, this still represented an actual increase to 2.4 million families. The strength of this social class is reflected in the fact that fully 60 percent were husband-wife families. In our view, this is at once the most important and vulnerable of all sectors of the class structure. It is not the underclass nor the middle class but the stable blue-collar working class that deserves the highest priority in public policy. A fortification and growth of this stratum would have two effects simultaneously. It would help to stem the downward flow into the underclass and resume the upward flow into the middle and upper classes.

A modicum of public attention is now being given to the black middle class. It is as though this is another discovery of "the new Negro." Middle-class families are those with family incomes between $25,000 and $50,000 in 1983 dollars. They also tend to be highly educated, with a majority having education beyond high school, and to occupy professional, technical, and managerial occupations. They also tend to be dual-earner families.

Indeed, as Harriette McAdoo has pointed out, black middle-class husbands often maintain their level not only by having a second working person in the family but a second job as well, generally on a part-time basis.

While the proportion of middle-class families doubled during the decade of the 1960s from 12 percent to 25 percent, reaching an all-time high of 29 percent in 1978, there has been a decline in recent years. While the percentages have been declining, the actual number of middle-class families has expanded from 1.1 million families in 1969 to 1.5 million by 1983. And, by 1986, there were 1.9 million black families in this sector.

The black middle class also tends to have a high proportion of husband-wife families. Thus, an overwhelming majority of 83 percent of families in this sector were husband-wife families. Further, working wives and mothers are the keys to the viability of the black middle class. Fully 78 percent of these families have working wives, more than any of the other four socioeconomic sectors. Moreover, the financial contribution black women make to the family income is increasing and is substantially higher than that in white families.

Finally, at the peak of the African-American social-class structure is a small and growing black upper class. This sector is completely overlooked in most studies of black families, in part because it is so small. Still, an accurate understanding of African-American family life requires a recognition that this stratum has significance far beyond its numbers.

Upper-class families are those with median family incomes ranging upward from $50,000 to above $200,000 in 1983 dollars and who possess substantial wealth and economic power. It is not the absolute income, however, but the accumulated wealth that distinguishes the black upper class. Wealth or net worth is measured as total assets owned minus total debts owed. Overall, the average black-family wealth is less than 10 percent of average white-family wealth, nearly $4,000 for black families and $40,000 for whites. Even among middle-class black families, it is $18,000, constituting only one-third of the wealth of similar white families. However, among a few black families, the accumulated wealth rises distinctly above the white median. Thus, some 12 percent of black families have accumulated wealth above $50,000. Moreover, some 4 percent of all black families have accumulated wealth above $100,000, a position they share with 24 percent of white American families. These families tend to be headed by highly educated parents in middle- and high-status public and private occupations and business ownership. They also tend to involve a high proportion of two working partners in the labor force.

For those African-American families who have been able to accumulate substantial financial assets, the principal instruments are home ownership, real estate, automobiles, and savings accounts. Relatively little has been invested in business ownership, stocks, and bonds.

A very important source of support for the socialization of black children with pioneering role models is provided by the small group of black families who have moved to the top of the socioeconomic structure by the ownership and management of their own business enterprises. Each year, *Black Enterprise* magazine profiles the black families owning the largest 100 black-owned businesses. Few more inspiring role models of upper-class blacks can be found than the John H. Johnson family of Chicago, the George A. Russell family of Atlanta, or the Earl Graves family of New York.

These families are not likely to be as well-known as some other upper-class families. Nevertheless, they are important role models, especially in a society that places such high values on private enterprise and in areas where blacks need a great deal of encouragement. These families at the top of the socioeconomic structure are few in number, but the important point is that their tribes are increasing.

In 1969, there were some 143,000 families in this black upper-class stratum comprising a tiny 3 percent of all African-American families in the nation. Half of all these families had working wives, and the other half were more traditional with husbands in the work-force while wives and mothers were full-time homemakers. By 1983, this stratum had expanded to embrace some 267,000 families comprising 4 percent of all African-American families in the nation. This small sector of African-American families had expanded so rapidly during the 1980s that by 1986, they comprised 9 percent of the total and included some 624,000 families.

One reason for looking at social-class stratification is that it helps to show diversity in other dimensions of life including family structure. Thus, among the black upper class, an overwhelming 96 percent are husband-wife families. At a time when it was commonly asserted that 42 percent of all African-American families were female-headed families, it is of some consequence to note that only 4 percent of the black upper class, 17 percent of the middle class, and 40 percent of nonpoor working-class families consisted of single parents. Only among the two poor sectors, the working poor and the nonworking poor, did single-parent families constitute the majority. Briefly, the impact of social class on family status is suggested by Table 5.1.

In sum, socioeconomic class stratification is an important, if often overlooked, dimension of African-American family life. A holistic approach that understands the full range of socioeconomic statuses in the black community can teach all of us the following lessons crucial to the well-being of black families.

First, it can teach all of us and our black children and youth that there is, indeed, room at the top and all along the socioeconomic ladder in legitimate enterprises to challenge and channel all their talents, interests, and abilities. They can achieve their aspirations in a wide variety of fields and be rewarded for them if they have the talent, the interest, and the help that they need.

TABLE 5.1. African-American Social Class and Family Structure

Class	Married-Couple	Single-Parent	Family Structure Working-Wife
Upper Class	96%	04%	50%
Middle Class	83%	17%	78%
Working Class (Nonpoor)	60%	40%	45%
Working Class (Poor)	33%	67%	33%
Underclass (Nonworking Poor)	25%	75%	25%

Source: U.S. Bureau of the Census.

Second, a view of the entire socioeconomic structure can teach us that individual achievement is not incompatible with stable family development, but, instead, they often go hand-in-hand.

Third, we learn from reflecting on these successful families that a remarkable concomitant to financial, occupational, and educational success is the ability to make a contribution to others.

These, then, are insights we gain from understanding African-American family diversity that we would never appreciate from examining the black underclass alone.

CONCLUSION

In sum, then, generalizations about African-American family patterns often degenerate into stereotypes because they fail to put these families in a holistic perspective. They fail to understand the complexity and diversity of these families. In their legitimate concern with single-parent families, generalizations fail to appreciate the extent of black family structural diversity. In their focus on the underclass at the bottom of the socioeconomic scale, they ignore the working class, the middle class, and the upper class. In their focus on adolescent behavior, including school failure and teen parenting, they ignore important dimensions of the life cycle at younger and older age ranges. Finally, in an often myopic focus on the family as an institution, they ignore its interdependence with the institutional structure of the black community and with the systems of the larger society.

There is an urgent need in African-American family studies for a broader view as urged by DuBois a century ago. Such an approach will help us understand these families better. It will help us to see more clearly their connection with other families. More important, it will help us to fashion sounder theories and sounder policies to enhance the structure and the functioning of these families.

REFERENCES

Billingsley, Andrew. (1993). *Climbing Jacob's ladders: The enduring legacy of African-American families*: New York: Simon and Schuster.

McAdoo, Harriette P. (1978). "Factors related to stability in upwardly mobile Black families," *Journal of Marriage and the Family*, 40(4):761-778.

Chapter 6

From the Tenement Class to the Dangerous Class to the Underclass: Blaming Women for Social Problems

Mimi Abramovitz

The Bible says the poor will always be with us, but does not say why. Since then, observers have tried to determine both the causes of social problems and their persistence. The mainstream explanations fall into two key groups: behavioral analyses, which attribute social problems to defective character, and individual dysfunctions and structural theories, which link poverty to malfunctioning societal institutions and problems in the political economy. The structural analysis lost ground in the mid-1980s and is out of vogue in today's policy debates, which are driven instead by a theory of the underclass that blames poverty on the behavior and values of the poor.

The focus here is on the behavioral theories of poverty. They merit careful critique given their long history, current popularity, and strong influence on social work practice and social welfare policy. For example, today's behavioral explanations of poverty are being used to justify meanspirited welfare reforms such as limiting welfare to two years, denying aid to children born on welfare, docking the welfare grant if children supported by Aid to Families with Dependent Children (AFDC) are too truant or do not get their shots, and fingerprinting welfare applicants.

The theories tend to become more popular in hard times when economic crises indict the market economy for its inability to pro-

---

This chapter was originally published in *Feminist Practice in the 21st Century*, ©1995, National Association of Social Workers, Inc. Reprinted by permission.

vide enough jobs or income. Such theories also do well in disruptive times as when rapid changes in women's roles appear to undermine patriarchal arrangements. By explaining away mounting social problems in individual rather than systemic terms, the theories protect the system from itself. Also, these theories favor punitive programs and less government spending.

The behavioral theories of poverty also merit review because their emphasis on intergenerational poverty often blames women when things go wrong. Long before "dependency" became a household word, families were blamed for transmitting undesirable values and behaviors from one generation to the next. Given the gender division of labor characterized by male breadwinning and female homemaking, this thinking implicitly and regularly blames mothers. Fueled by the nation's historic and deep-seated distrust of poor women's capacity to properly raise their children—from the morally defective family to the schizophrenigenic mother to the welfare queen—twentieth-century behavioral theories have been deeply misogynist. From Social Darwinism and eugenics before World War I to psychoanalysis in the 1940s and 1950s, to the "culture of poverty," social science has portrayed poor women as breeders of the "tenement classes," the "dangerous classes," and most recently, the "underclass." Only the means of transmission have changed over time from moral contagion to genetic transmission to psychological internalization to cultural dissemination.

MORAL CONTAGION

The early behavioral theories of poverty dwelled on moral contagion. They first gained a foothold in the mid-1800s when the emerging market economy dislodged people from the land but could not steadily employ all those ready and willing to work. Ignoring the changing economy, social observers attributed rising poverty rates to moral deficiencies of individuals transmitted from one generation to another in the homes of the tenement class, "whose lazy and ignorant members—drunkards, gamblers, spendthrifts, prostitutes, sinners, and foreigners—lacked moral feeling and sense of shame."[1] To officialdom, slum life meant "something wrong at home." Poor children were cursed "not by poverty principally, but by the ungoverned appetite, bad habits, and vices of their parents," who in the view of the experts lacked self-control, thrift, sobriety, and sexual restraint.[2] If white homes were the "moral pests of society," to officialdom, African Americans, most of whom were still slaves, "had no sense of family life at all" and needed to "be made faithful to the marriage bond and taught their sense of ancestry."[3]

The moral contagion theory implicitly condemned mothers for the inferior quality of life that early industrialization offered to the poor. The practice of blaming social problems on improper home life instead of the dynamics of capitalist development became credible, in part, because the new vision of middle-class family life made the normal patterns of the poor and the working class appear deviant. The separation of household and market production that accompanied industrialization generated a new definition of both gender roles and the home. Men went to work in the factories, women focused exclusively on family caretaking, and the home became a private refuge shielding the family from the outside dangers of corruption and commercialism.[4]

The lives of the poor did not fit this idealized image in the eyes of the middle class. To them the poor lived in crowded neighborhoods filled with teeming streets, ramshackle tenements without bathtubs and private toilets, and unattended children. In contrast to the notion of the home as private refuge, these conditions were "evidence" of parental neglect, family disintegration, and pervasive social pathology rather than an expected outcome of life in overcrowded apartments and communities.[5] Parents who sent their children to work, left them unsupervised, or gave them "excessive" responsibility for the home were deemed "cruel" by The Society for the Prevention of Cruelty to Children.[6] Charity workers depicted working-class mothers, especially if single or employed, as a subhuman species: bestially drunk, abusive, indifferent as well as unwomanly, and neglectful, if not dangerous to future generations. To the middle class, poor families and neighborhoods were breeding grounds of degeneracy, the "parent[s] of constant disorder and the nurser[ies] of vice."[7]

These perceptions of the poor dictated the preferred remedies. Disdainful of the homes of the poor, the mid-nineteenth century reformers hoped to prevent "moral contagion" by cutting relief (viewed as pauperizing people), removing children from their parents' care, resocializing mothers, and seeking child support from the fathers. They also began to place the poor in workhouses, orphanages, asylums, prisons, and other institutions. These policies applied largely to whites. Until the end of the Civil War, most African-American women were enslaved, treated as property, forced to work the land, and forced to breed future slaves. The inhumane practices of slavery were followed by Jim Crow. Such practices were justified by the prevailing belief in racial inferiority.

GENETIC TRANSMISSION

Between the Civil War and World War I, rapid industrialization, urbanization, and immigration created new and deeper social problems that required explanation. Social Darwinism and eugenics, the dominant social theories of the day, produced new intergenerational transmission explanations of social problems focused on genes and heredity. Social Darwinism transformed Darwin's theory of biological evolution based on natural selection and survival of the fittest, into a theory of social selection in which the struggle of economic survival separated the "fit" and "unfit." The eugenics movement held that acquired traits were inherited.[8] Both became embedded in public opinion and social policy; once again, women were blamed. For example, a well-known report on the poor houses stated that poorhouse inmates had "inherited their distaste of work and their fondness for drink from their pauper parents."[9] Studies of immigrant families such as ones by Jukes (1877) and Killikaks (1912) concluded that feeble-mindedness was inherited and responsible for spawning endless generations of deviants and "defectives."[10] A highly praised 1910 study of blacks insisted that "in [their] home life the Negro is filthy, careless and indecent, . . . as destitute of morals as many of the lower animals, . . . [and with] little knowledge of the sanctity of the home or marital relations."[11]

Both Social Darwinism and eugenics held that in a competitive capitalist environment, those with courage, enterprise, good training, intelligence, and perseverance naturally rose to the top while the physically, morally, or mentally weak rightfully fell to the bottom. They equated the fit with the rich, native born, and whites and the unfit with the poor, foreign born, and nonwhite. Some even wanted to stop the unfit from reproducing.[12]

The belief in the intergenerational transmission of deviant behavior through "bad" genes reflected deep nativist fears that a flood of immigrants threatened the purity and integrity of the native-born racial stock as well as that the undesirables propagated by immigrants resulted in lower intelligence, slowed down the economy, and undermined the nation. If left unchecked, they would overrun the "human" race. Social Darwinism and eugenics also supported white domination as naturally ordained and fueled the period's virulent racism, which eventually legalized segregation after the Civil War.[13] Given the gender division of labor, hereditarian theories by definition implicated women. As the biological and social reproducers of the next generation, who else transmitted deviant behavior? Nativists linked their fears of race suicide to women's changing roles. They protested increased female employment and the falling birth rate among native-born college-educated women. Theodore Roosevelt actually accused native-born white women who refused to have large families of being "criminals against the race."[14]

While glorifying motherhood, the reformers condemned women who did not measure up to the ideal. Not only were "degraded women" the visible links in the direful chain of hereditary, pauperism and disease," but reformers asked should the "diseased and viscous" be allowed to reproduce?" Pointing to the practice of lifetime incarceration for the incurably insane, Josephine Shaw Lowell, a charity leader, asked, "Why should we not also prevent the transmission of moral insanity [e.g., women arrested for a misdemeanor, and women who gave birth to a second out-of-wedlock child] as fatal as that of the mind?"[15]

Once again behavioral theories of social problems drove social policy toward family breakup and less relief. Charity reformers hoped to stop the spread of "dependence" from one generation to the next "by snapping the bonds between pauper parents and their children." Poorhouse superintendents heard in 1870 that the "surest way of correcting the great evil of hereditary pauperism was to separate children from their parents."[16] Others were warned that society neglects its duty "when it allows a child to remain with a parent that persistently teaches it beggary and crime."[17]

In addition to favoring family breakup, officials closed down public relief offices in major cities on the ground that relief created social problems. They institutionalized more of the "feebleminded" and called for immigration quotas, marriage restrictions, and compulsory sterilization. By the end of World War I, immigrants and the poor filled state institutions, and by 1917, sterilization laws existed in twenty-five states.[18]

The eugenics movement finally lost ground to new scientific findings, its inherent racism, and its use by Hitler in the 1930s, but the deep distrust of poor women's ability to properly socialize their children persisted. The idea of the intergenerational transmission of deviant values and behaviors by women reappeared in new forms.

PSYCHOLOGICAL INTERNALIZATION

Twentieth-century theorists transformed theories of the intergenerational transmission of undesirable values and behavior from a biological to a psychological event and extended the antiwoman analysis to the middle class. Having rejected moral and genetic contagion as the transmitter of social problems, new theories emphasized psychological transmission through childrearing and the mother-child tie.[19]

In the early twentieth century, social scientists disparaged traditional mother love as the basis for properly reared children in favor of "scientific motherhood." Mother love came to be viewed as too sentimental, as a "dangerous instrument" that spoiled children and encouraged them to be dependent, undisciplined, and nonconforming. Such children would not mesh with the rationality, efficiency, and order in all spheres of life now demanded by the rapidly industrializing economy. The stern practice of "scientific mothering"—strict feeding and sleeping schedules, early toilet training, minimal maternal affection—was intended to instill the habits of regularity needed to make future workers obedient, punctual, and good citizens. Drawing on Watson's psychological behaviorism, scientific mothering would also prevent laziness, delinquency, class antagonisms, and poverty.[20]

Scientific mothering implicitly linked irregular mothering to family and social problems, but poor and working-class women were especially suspect and vulnerable to failing the tests of scientific motherhood. While some introduced parent education classes to help poor women, Watson and others argued that "no one should have a child until she could afford to give the child a room of its own," and suggested that "poor and working-class women should not have children at all."[21]

Scientific mothering was eventually superseded by mental hygiene theory, but mothers continued to be blamed when things went wrong. According to mental hygiene theory, the normal personality depended on the quality of emotional ties in the home, rather than discipline and control. Families with satisfying relationships produced well-adjusted children who could accept frustration and deprivation, external authority, and one's station in life. Poor parenting (read: mothering) led to maladjusted or deviant behavior and social problems. In addition to standardized tests of normality, the mental hygiene movement supported mental health clinics and parent education services.[22]

In the 1930s new theories urged more responsive parenting and flexible rather than rigid childrearing. The shift to more permissive childrearing coincided with rise of mass-produced goods and services after World War I and the intensification of the consumerism. If Americans had to follow the industrial clock before World War I, postwar business wanted them to replace spartan habits of frugality for indulgence and self-gratification, on which consumption depended. Previously suppressed impulses now were encouraged as healthy for personality development and the wider economy.[23]

Freud's theory that undue repression of children's needs could result in lifelong psychological damage fit right in as did Arnold Gesell's theory that feeding, weaning, and toilet training be set by the child's demands and follow set stages. Each theory posited an ideal mother whose personality, self-sacrifice, and unconditional love would assure that she did not produce psychologically damaged children prone to deviant behavior. Gessell's ideal mother created self-determined children by following the child's lead, never disrupting the phase. Psychoanalysis posited a biologically based maternal instinct, self-sacrificing mothers who achieved fulfillment by serving others, and children who needed a full-time mother who would play, stimulate, and nurture their offspring; encourage their impulses; and provide unconditional love. To want anything else was abnormal for a woman.[24]

Reflecting this thinking and fueled by women's changing roles, mother blaming reached new heights during World War II (1941-1945). The war pushed poverty to the back burner and men to the frontline and created consumer shortages. It also pulled massive numbers of married women into labor force. Hoping to stem the wartime changes in gender roles, experts translated public fears about women's changing roles into questions about women's ability to raise children. Wartime hardships and postwar social problems were increasingly blamed on mothering.[25]

When more than two million men were rejected for service for psychological reasons, the armed service's psychiatric consultant accused "America's traditional, sweet, doting, self-sacrificing mom" of having "failed in the elementary mother function of weaning offspring emotionally as well as physically." Philip Wylie's 1942 bestselling *A Generation of Vipers* blamed overpowering women and "momism" for psychological and emotional immaturity in children.[26]

After the war, fears about the decline of the traditional family were fueled by rising rates of female employment, divorce, nonmarital births, illegal abortions, juvenile delinquency, and homosexuality. Experts chastised white middle-class fathers as nighttime residents and weekend guests, but they most often dammed the suburban family as child centered and female dominated. Two negative but contradictory images emerged: the overprotective, over-involved, overpowering mother and the depriving, rejecting mother who scarred her children and society by working outside of the home or having interests of her own.

The widely read book *The Modern Women: The Lost Sex* (1947) concluded that only half of America's mothers were "healthy, fully maternal mothers who merely loved their children. The other half were unhealthy—rejecting, overprotective, or dominating." The authors, Lundberg and Farnham, attributed most neuroses in Western civilization to the unwomanly drive to power that festered in the home until women destroyed the people around them.[27]

Psychoanalytic theory maligned full-time mothers, calling them "aggressive," hostile, and overbearing. With more white middle-class wives restlessly confined to the home, experts began to argue that mothers hurt their children by subconsciously displacing their own frustrations and needs for independence and achievement onto them. If full-time mothers put children and society in harm's way, working mothers were even worse. Based on his studies of the withdrawn condition of institutionalized World War II orphans, John Bolby wrongly concluded that the negative symptoms were due to the maternal deprivation that could occur whenever the home lacked a full-time mother. This version of the intergenerational theory of social problems claimed that whether in their own homes or out of them, "maternally deprived children" are a source of social infection as real and serious as the carriers of diphtheria and typhoid, thus calling for a mass public health campaign to detect cases of deprivation.[28]

To control the "dangerous trends" that threatened the patriarchal family, postwar mental health experts in all fields advised working mothers to quit their jobs and return to their natural state of motherhood. Backed by Bowlby's 1950s studies of maternal deprivation, Freudian theory of female sexuality, and sociologist Talcott Parson's one breadwinner/one homemaker nuclear family model, the experts stressed the mother-child bond, accused working mothers of child deprivation and unnatural female instincts, and blamed them for a vast array of problems ranging from bedwetting to juvenile delinquency to schizophrenia.

In the words of Betty Friedan, who wrote from the 1940s to the early 1960s:

> It was suddenly discovered that the mother could be blamed for everything. In every case history of the troubled child; alcoholic, suicidal, schizophrenic, psychopathic, neurotic adult; impotent, homosexual male; frigid, promiscuous female; ulcerous, asthmatic, and otherwise disturbed American could be found a mother. A frustrated, repressed, disturbed, martyred, never satisfied, unhappy woman. A rejecting, overprotecting, dominating mother.[29]

This psychological analysis of social problems was directed largely to the white middle class, but blaming women's psyche for social problems also trickled down to the white and black working class and poor. Some social workers, I am sorry to say, held that poverty and the need for relief stemmed from deeply rooted childhood dependency wishes and that rising crime, mental illness, and suicide was due to women's employment and inadequate parenting. Review of child protection records indicate that the previously neglectful parent became the neurotic or pathological mother.[30] Single mothers were seen as "fallen" women raising "illegitimate" children in "unstable" families or "broken" homes especially if they were black.[31] Lesbians of all classes were simply sick.

The negative postwar images of African-American women were laced with degrading racist stereotypes as well as a negative view of employed women. Black women were Sapphires—the overbearing wife of Kingfish on *Amos 'n' Andy*—or castrating matriarchs who ruled the female-headed household, overpowered their men, emasculated their sons, and transmitted low social and moral standards to family members.[32] Echoing century-old racist myths, black women became the hypersexual Jezebel or the warm and simple black Mammy possessed of a natural affection that made her an ideal caretaker of white children.[33]

The argument that pathological behavior is "transmitted" from parent to child through the mother's impaired psyche persists to this day. Perhaps it was coincidental that natural childbirth, breast feeding and the theory of maternal-child bonding came into vogue in the 1970s at the height of the women's movement. Despite mixed evidence on bonding, one pediatric expert declared that infants who do not bond properly can become terrorists. A 1980s *New York Times Magazine* article titled "Mothers: Tired of Taking the Rap" concluded that "[m]others have been made the cause of everything from colic to mass murder."[34]

Mother-child relationships cannot be dismissed as an important factor in shaping children's adult personality. However, singling out mothers and ignoring the role of fathers and of wider social conditions leads to a highly distorted view of social problems and sanctions punitive social work practices and social polices, especially those targeted at women.

CULTURAL DISSEMINATION

With the "rediscovery of poverty" in the 1960s, a new behavioral theory of poverty reappeared with its own presumptions about the intergenerational transmission of "destructive" values and behavior.

This time the source of contagion was a defective culture, not defective morals, bad genes, or a distorted psyche. Based on his anthropological studies of Mexican and Puerto Rican barrios in the early 1960s, Oscar Lewis posited the existence of a culture of poverty—a set of values and behaviors that prevented children from using the few opportunities that come their way and thus tended to perpetuate itself from generation to generation. To Lewis, the culture of poverty was a means by which the poor adapted to their marginalized position in a class-stratified society. It was a by-product of capitalism.[35]

When neoconservatives such as Edward Banfield and Daniel Moynihan adopted the Culture of Poverty theory, they stressed its behavioral over its structural analysis and heightened the misogyny. Moynihan's 1965 report, *The Negro Family: A Case for National Action,* blamed female-headed households for the problems faced by the black community, although at the time, the overwhelming majority of black families contained two parents. Moynihan claimed that mother-only families deprived their children of a male role model and a proper authority figure, trapped their families in a "tangle of pathology," and created a cycle of poverty.[36] Any social problems found in the black community stemmed from the structure of the black family, not poverty or racism. To some it was no accident that this victim-blaming analysis of black families resurfaced just when the increasingly militant Civil Rights movement attracted more public attention to racial injustice.[37]

The Culture of Poverty theory, which receded in the storm of protests unleashed by Moynihan's report, has been resurrected by the currently popular "theory of the underclass."[38] Social scientists describe the underclass today as a socially isolated segment of the poor, living in disorganized neighborhoods characterized not only by high rates of crime, hustling, drug abuse, school dropouts, and joblessness, but also high rates of teenage pregnancy, female-headed households, out-of-wedlock births, and welfare use.[39]

You do not have to listen too hard to hear the message that crime, drug use, and school dropouts are among the "tangle of pathologies" that are transmitted from one generation to another by women (of color) heading families without a male at the helm. The message is clear: Welfare mothers are no different from drug users and criminals.

As with earlier intergenerational theories of poverty, the under-class theory has become firmly embedded in the current social dogma, where it fuels support for increasingly punitive social poli-cies for poor women. During the 1980s, the theory sanctioned social programs cutbacks, which threw thousands of women off AFDC, allowed their benefits to erode by 40 percent, and made it more difficult for them to get housing, food stamps, Medicaid, and needed social services. Today, the underclass theory drives mean-spirited welfare reforms that use government dollars to regulate the lives of women and sink women and children deeper into poverty. Both Clinton's Welfare Reform Plan and numerous state initiatives are grounded in the negative stereotype of welfare mothers as culturally adrift welfare queens who prefer welfare to work, live high on the hog, cheat the government, and have kids for money. Likewise, AFDC is accused of removing women from the labor force, causing families to break up, encouraging nonmarital births, and otherwise inducing irresponsible behavior.

Despite the lack of research support for a relationship between welfare and a women's work and family choices, the welfare reformers continue to press for workfare, wedfare, learnfare, and healthfare programs—programs which presume that undesirable values and behavior are transmitted from deviant mother to child. To "break the cycle," workfare and Clinton's two-year cap requires women to go to work or face reduced benefits; learnfare docks the checks of welfare mothers whose children miss school too often; healthfare lowers the grant to mothers whose children are not immu-nized. Most controversial of all are the efforts to control the repro-duction by poor women through the child exclusion or family cap, which denies aid to children born while the family is on the rolls. Some states also want to make Norplant, the contraceptive implant, a condition of aid, and some judges have tried to make it a condition of parole. Charles Murray and the family values camp have recently resurrected the once-discredited language of "illegitimacy," defined it as the prime cause of poverty, crime, and violence, and called for ending it by eliminating all AFDC, Food Stamps, and housing sub-sidies. These proposals, along with Murray's new book, *The Bell Curve*, echo the eugenic movement's fear of breeding by the poor. Can forced sterilization be far behind?

CONCLUSION: WHAT THE FUTURE HOLDS

Conservative theories of poverty, which blame social and economic problems on women rather than the profit-oriented decisions of business and the state, have once again captured the social policy agenda; such policies recommend fixing the poor instead of the economy. The question is why? Blaming women for social distress is easy in a society that dislikes the poor, women, and persons of color. Blaming women also upholds work and family norms—especially when social policy such as welfare reform is used to discipline those women who do not live up to the idealized version of womanhood. Penalizing husbandless women on AFDC, for example, sends a message to all women about what awaits those who fail "to play by the rules." Finally, blaming poverty and other social problems on the intergenerational transmission of deviant values and behavior through the home is one of the many tricks used to deflect attention from the real underlying causes: poverty, sexism, racism, and inequality.

What about the social work profession? Where does it stand in all this? How have we been seduced or coopted by behavioral explanations of social problems? Have terms such as "underclass," "welfare dependency," and the "culture of poverty" crept into our personal and professional language? Do we understand that when we use this language, we become hostage to the negative metaphors about women, race, and poverty that these words convey. Accepting them we risk letting our own behavior and thoughts be shaped by their victim-blaming misogynist and racist definitions of people, poverty, or society and buy into the current justification for cutting the welfare state.

What can social work do? First, we need to identify, reclaim, and reinstate the profession's long-standing liberal and radical heritage. This means—among other things—basing our work on structural not behavioral theories of poverty. Second, as a field populated by women workers and clients, we are well positioned to oppose victim-blaming rationales, to call for social policies that help rather than punish women, and to help unify women by making it clear that an injury to one is an injury to all.

Third, we can think about a new basis for social policy that will bring people together. To this end, we might promote social policies that address the mounting caregiving crisis. Regardless of race, class, or marital status, most women can no longer carry out the family maintenance task assigned to them without additional supports from men, employers, and the state. Since the mid-1970s changes in women's role, the diversification family structures, and the limits of the economy intensified the need for family supports. At the very same time, they actively disinvest in the welfare state. As a result there are few two-earner professional couples, working-class households, and single mothers who do not worry about providing care to children, sick family members, and aging parents and about getting meals cooked, food bought, and homes cleaned.

While the most affluent women can buy the services they need, the overwhelming majority of women must suffer the stress of the double day. Very poor and homeless people worry if they will eat and where they will sleep tomorrow. Today's punitive campaign for welfare reform should alarm us all. It obscures the fact that the plight of the single mother on welfare is but caretaking crises faced by all women.

What can we do? In addition to watching our language and fighting for progressive change, social workers can join forces with those women in struggle who refuse to take the blame, the punishment, or the coercion of welfare reform lying down. This includes welfare mothers who have begun to organize and protest across the nation and are receiving support from major feminist groups such as National Organization of Women (NOW) and The Bertha Capen Reynolds Society. Both groups have invited the President of the National Welfare Rights union to address their national convention and made welfare reform an organizational priority. These political actions are critical. The historical record shows that the "powers that be" rarely act and social policy rarely changes for the better unless pressured from below.

NOTES

1. Boyer, P. (1978). *Urban masses and moral order in America 1820-1920.* Cambridge, MA: Harvard University Press, p. 90.

2. Brace, C. L. (1880/1967). *The dangerous classes.* Montclair, NJ: Patterson Smith; Boyer, p. 39; Scott, D. M., and Wishy, B. (1982). *America's families: A documentary history.* New York: Harper and Row, p. 384; Stansell, C. (1986).

City of women: Sex and class in New York 1789-1860. Urbana: University of Illinois Press, p. 202.

3. Fitzhugh (1866) quoted in Gutman, H. C. (1983). Persistent myths about the Afro-American family. In M. Gordon (ed.), *The American family in social-historical perspective*. New York: St. Martin's Press, pp. 450-481.

4. Mathaie, J. A. (1982). *An economic history of women in America: Women's work, the sexual division of labor and the development of capitalism*. New York: Schoken Books; Scott and Wispy; Ryan, M. (1975). *Womanhood in America: From colonial times to the present*. New York: New Viewpoints.

5. Stansell, p. 202.

6. Gordon, L. (1988). *Heroes of their own lives: The politics and history of family violence*. New York: Penguin Books.

7. Stansell, p. 202.

8. Ehrenreich, J. H. (1985). *The altruistic imagination: A history of social work and social policy in the United States*. Ithaca: Cornell University Press; Hofstadter, R. (1955). *Social Darwinism in American thought*. Boston: Beacon Press; Katz, M. B. (1986). *In the shadow of the poorhouse: A social history of welfare in America*. New York: Basic Books.

9. Katz, pp. 86-87.

10. Gordon, L.; Katz; Solinger, R. (1992). *Wake up little Susie: Single pregnancy and race relations before Roe v. Wade*. New York: Routledge; Trattner, W. I. (1989). *From poor law to welfare state: A history of social welfare in America*. New York: The Free Press.

11. Odum, H. (1910). *Social and mental traits of the Negro: Research into the basic conditions of the Negro race in southern towns*. New York.

12. Ehrenreich; Hofstadter; Katz.

13. Allen, R. (1975). *Reluctant reformers: Racism and social reform movements in the United States*. New York: Anchor Books; Hofstadter.

14. Ladd-Taylor, M. (1987). "Mother-work, ideology, public policy, and the mother's movement." Unpublished PhD dissertation. Yale University, p. 2.

15. Lowell, J. S. (1879). One means of preventing pauperism. *Proceedings of the sixth annual conference of charities*. Boston, June, pp. 189-200.

16. Katz, p. 107.

17. Ambramovitz, M. (1992, fourth printing). *Regulating the lives of women: Social welfare policy from colonial times to the present*. Boston: South End Press, p. 153.

18. Katz; Lubove, R. (1965). *The professional altruist: The emergence of social work as a career 1880-1930*. Cambridge, MA: Harvard University Press.

19. Ehrenreich, B., and English, D. (1979). *For her own good: 100 years of the experts' advice to women*. New York: Anchor Books.

20. Ehrenreich; Ladd-Taylor; Mintz, S., and Kellog, S. (1988). *Domestic revolutions: A social history of American family life*. New York: The Free Press; Scott and Wispy.

21. Ehrenreich and English, p. 205.

22. Ehrenreich; Mathaie.

23. Ehrenreich and English; Ladd-Taylor; Mintz and Kellog; Ryan.

24. Ehrenreich and English; Ladd-Taylor; Mintz and Kellog; Ryan.

25. Mintz and Kellog.

26. Ehrenreich and English; Mintz and Kellog.

27. Mathaie.

28. Ehrenreich and English.

29. Mintz and Kellog.

30. Gordon.

31. Solinger.

32. Collins, P. H. (1990). *Black feminist thought, knowledge, consciousness, and the politics of empowerment*. London: HarperCollins Academic; Gilkes, C. T. (1983). From slavery to social welfare: Racism and the control of black women. In A. Swerdlow and H. Lessinger (eds.), *Class, race and sex: The dynamics of control*. Boston: G. K. Hall.

33. Ehrenreich and English; Solinger.

34. Smith, J. M. (1990, June 10). Mothers: Tired of taking the rap. *The New York Times Magazine*, 2-33, 38, p. 32.

35. Lewis, O. (1966, October). The culture of poverty. *Scientific American* 215, pp. 19-25; Lewis, O. (1961). *The children of Sanchez*. New York: Random House; Wilson, W. J. (1985). Cycles of deprivation and the underclass debate. *Social Service Review*, 56(4), pp. 541-559.

36. Moynihan, D. P. (1965). *The Negro family: The case for national action*. Washington, DC: Government Printing Office.

37. Gresham, J. H., and Wilkerson, M. B. (1989). The politics of family in America. *The Nation*, July 24/31, pp. 116-120.

38. Wilson, W. J. (1985). Cycles of deprivation and the underclass debate. *Social Service Review*, 56(4), pp. 541-559.

39. Mincy, R., Sawhill, I. V., and Wolff, D. A. (1990). The underclass: Definition and Measurement. *Science*, 248, pp. 450-453; Ricketts, E. R., and Sawhill, I. V. (1988). Defining and measuring the underclass. *Journal of Policy Analysis and Management*, 7(2), pp. 316-325.

Chapter 7

Health and Human Services for Profit

Joseph L. Vigilante

PURPOSE

The purpose of this chapter is to comment on the history and current plans and policies concerning the privatization of human services, with special attention to the conceivable effects on social development goals. The discussion draws heavily on Martin Rein's concept of a "value-critical" methodology[1] and considers the possible realization of Rein's anticipation of a change in assessing social policy from an "efficiency" orientation to a "value orientation,"[2] an epistemological shift whose time has (perhaps) come.

Opportunities to achieve the elusive goals of civil rationality are seriously hampered as our era ignores or rejects established civilizing beliefs about mutual human responsibilities for mutual caring. The strained relationships between political, social, and economic forces and human values, which have led to the decline of the welfare state, have contributed to the concomitant rise of the free market as a milieu for delivering human social and health services. I shall discuss the likely results of this initiative and the feasibility of a radical *epistemological* paradigm (Martin Rein's value-critical method), which is admittedly a long-shot solution for the current crisis of social development.

THE CARING SOCIETY

The policy decision implied by the 1994 election of the conservative Republican Congress is that the *caring society* in the form of the welfare state has been a failure—perhaps more accurately, an unacceptable burden on government. This burden is described by Congressional executioners in terms of taxes, the national debt, and the moral behavior of the poor. Newt Gingrich's "Contract with America" and ensuing federal legislation have simulated or permitted a series of policy decisions at the local, state, and federal levels which supplant the "caring" paradigm of the welfare state with a market paradigm that treats social caring as a business.[3] This frame of reference suggests the availability of human services as a hostage for profit, a drastic reversal of the Western humanitarian tradition. The effort to place social policy in the marketplace begs an understanding of the *meaning* and the *means* of social caring—how to preserve and enhance rational, civil, and just human relationships while ensuring against the social risks posed by industrialization and technological advance.

All forms of postagrarian free societies—industrial, postindustrial, modern, postmodern—have fashioned a variety of methods for pursuing goals for rational living. Peter Drucker,[4] for example, has identified two dominant and separate streams of social organization in the United States: the market economy and the political/social system he calls the "polity." We seem to believe that stable and free social systems can be achieved through combinations of guaranteed individual freedoms and selected social controls that are mutually dependent on the economic and political community. Human services have been institutionalized necessities between two sectors (business and government) as a means of protecting against the risks of socially handicapping conditions. Institutionally established human services are essential for the achievement of adequate levels of rational living, although their tenuous location between business and government in a third "voluntary" sector has threatened the purpose of protection against social risks.

In this modern period, technological and social change have stimulated the establishment of institutionalized human support systems. Human service institutions are the lubricant for the gears that drive advanced complex social and economic systems. Throughout the twentieth century, human services (both financial supports and personal social service entitlements) have been key elements in social development. These have been steadily expanding through government leadership in all developed nations, drawing much public attention as well as reluctant support from conservatives in recent years. However, conservative resistance in the United States has been shifted from "quiet stonewalling" to aggressive attacks since the Republican Congressional victory of 1995.

The specter of the welfare state had been perceived intermittently by conservative elements as haunting the United States. The welfare state, conceived in Bismarck's Germany, was solidly established in England following World War II[5] and in most of Europe since. By the early 1980s, with the leadership of Reagan in Washington and Thatcher in London, the powers of conservatism entered into a modern holy alliance to exorcise the ghost. Political conservatives, fundamentalists, revivalists, and other special interests—from the Health Insurer's Association of America to the National Association of Manufacturers, to some extent the American Medical Association (and of course, Ross Perot)—have supported privatization of human services as a substitute with at least two advantages: government debt reduction and more efficient operation.

PRIVATIZING SOCIAL CARE

Massive privatization of human services promises to preserve or worsen the current unequal accessibility to essential human support services like day care, welfare, and health care, as well as to weaken a long-established commitment to the basic morals and human values of free societies. The principle of keeping human services outside the market economy had served as a reminder that mutual social obligations of the polity are basic conditions for rational moral living. Now, as the goals, values, and methods of the welfare state have been eroding,[6] public support for social caring wanes. The future of social care institutions is threatened as the third sector totters in precarious balance, and moral and social rationality lose public centrality. We observe the decline of community identity and civil behavior as the sale of human services for profit increases.

Privatization of human services is a momentous and enormous threat to human well-being. The contrary model, the welfare state, a *guaranteed universal provision of institutionalized human services*, provides at least two distinct linch pins for connecting industrialized society with civil rationality: (1) the remediation or prevention of ever-present social risks to individuals, families, and groups, and (2) the necessity for universal, broad community development, stressing human service programs and mutual community responsibility of the many for the few and the obligations of the few to the whole. In the welfare state model, these guarantees are not dependent on a market economy, which is necessarily subject to market variations; these are the business of the democratic governments of rational human beings.[7] An understanding of the impact of privatization on most human service professions requires careful attention to a range of macro and micro social, political, and economic forces (accompanied by neglect of human values) that are currently battering transitional societies throughout the world.

For the purposes of this analysis, the private sector is defined as organizations, corporations, and institutions in the "business" of *selling human services for profit. Nonprofit*, voluntary, publicly chartered institutions, often referred to as "private agencies," are *excepted*. The distinction between these two forms of service delivery is obscured by the word "private." In the context of equitable human service delivery, the operational word is "profit." While both are "private" compared to "public" tax-supported organizations, what is important is their difference in respect to seeking profits. I view as absurd the time-worn and usually unfounded allegation that nonprofit agencies earn profits from government contracts, given the oversight, control, monitoring, and audit systems utilized by governments at all levels, particularly in today's ultraconservative political/social climate. The practice of government funding of voluntary, nonprofit agencies to provide human services under a contract with government is hardly comparable to encouraging the sale of human services for profit in a competitive market. The distinction also draws attention to another inevitable result of corporate incursions into the human services; surplus profits can often be used as investment commodities to further multiply these profits. In this context one should not neglect a reference to the financing methods recommended to Congress for health care reform in the belated efforts to pass a national health program in 1994. Although a single-payer plan administered by the federal government would control profiting, this model was ignored by the Clinton administration as well as by most other proposals. All but one of the plans under consideration actually created opportunities for enormous profits on an unprecedented scale. Professor Burton C. DeLuca's letter (August 26, 1994) to *The New York Times* neatly sums up this particular scam:

> The least savory aspect of the proposed health care reform initiative is the prominence assigned to the five major private, for-profit health care insurers and their tag-along of lesser colleagues gathered in the Health Insurer's Association of America. This is the very crew whose practice in pursuit of their bottom line have [sic] helped to precipitate the crisis that reforms are intended to correct. They have turned the basic principle of insurance on its head; the wide sharing of risk so as to dilute excessive risk . . . Using the huge cash flows and "floats" of premium income, they have speculated in stock, bond, and money markets with the profits accruing to their bottom line and not to the lowering of premiums.

The escape from public responsibility to private profiting has been prompted by at least five important historical phenomena: (1) the increasing costs of human resource programs, (2) enormous national and world debts, (3) worldwide inflation not unrelated to monopolies in international trade, (4) a global swell of political conservatism, and (5) armament expenditures at the expense of social entitlements. These negative economic social forces gained strength steadily between 1960 and 1975. By 1980, the political successes of conservative parties provided the stimulus to begin dismantling welfare state structures in the United Kingdom, the United States, Sweden, Canada, West Germany, as well as other democratic nations, using rising costs of service and increases in national debts as a rationale. The rebirth of "welfare capitalism" in the United States began with Ronald Reagan's commitment to supply side economics,[8] drastic reductions in government spending for human services (including education), and an appeal to the private corporate sector to underwrite human services, couched in ideas reminiscent of Andrew Carnegie's Gospel of Wealth. In spite of next to no response from the corporate sector or the national financial community, eight years later George Bush's vaguely defined concept of voluntary social welfare through individuals, corporations, and philanthropic institutions, which he characteristically misnamed "a thousand points of light," was not taken seriously by many. These unsuccessful conservative initiatives represent blatant reversals of 100 years of the tradition of increasing government support of adequate, equitable, and accountable human services.

At the beginning of the twentieth century, business leaders such as Henry Ford had attempted to use the corporation as a "benevolent" provider of education, recreation, and other minor forms of "human service" to a usually passive population of low-paid immigrant workers. Even then, the price of corporate welfare was too high, and the economic collapse of 1929 demonstrated the futility of the private corporate sector as a healer of human deprivation. Privatization, the 1990s version of corporate welfare, is rekindled now by the attraction of *high profits*, rather than moral imperatives or the obligations of noblesse oblige. Nursing homes, health care, day care, and education seem to be the main targets for privatizing. *The New York Times* reported on October 5, 1994, that the entire school system of Hartford, Connecticut, was to be turned over to a private education management company for 50 percent of the profits, which it would earn through *savings*. Hartford was the company's sixth venture of this type and the sixth city in the United States to opt for privatized public education. By January of 1996, the contract was canceled as a result of the city's extreme disappointment with the program.

Our human services have always been understood as a *mixed* system. We have mixed polity functions with economic functions, but usually within balanced limits. We have had private, voluntary, nonprofit organizations delivering human services, even while the role of the government in social development steadily expanded. Today, the voluntary social service (not-for-profit) sector receives large amounts of government dollars (about $40 billion annually), signaling both the expanding need for human services and the reluctance of government to provide services, usually, if not exclusively, for partisan, political reasons.

THE DECLINE OF AMERICA'S WELFARE STATE

America's national welfare program was inaugurated with the Social Security Act in 1935. In 1975, the Title XX amendment to that law opened the door to a new partnership between government and *nonprofit agencies*. Most liberals welcomed this initiative during the 1970s as America's special version of the welfare state. The outcome has been paradoxical, for in a society in which big business currently (and properly) enjoys questionable credibility, it was (for government) a surprisingly easy giant step from supporting "nonprofits" to contracting with large, private, profit-driven corporations for human services in large quantities. To rationalize granting service contracts to private, profit-seeking corporations by citing the history of contracting with *nonprofit social agencies* is beyond absurdity, however typical this claim may be.

The privatization model currently operable in the corporate sector has already revealed serious limitations. Private corporate social services are usually "simple services" that are easily arranged and likely to be successful (not too much risk, if you please). It is clear that the central concern of corporations considering the human service market is whether it will eventually result in sufficient profit (a cost benefit criterion).[9] Specialized requirements in most welfare services lead to heightened risks that will reduce the number of firms that can bid on any given contract in the human services. Nelson notes that under these conditions, large firms of substandard quality emerge as dominant in the market. He predicts that with the complexity of the tasks required in human services, efforts to reduce costs will either compromise quality or reduce access,[10] as the history of social welfare has repeatedly demonstrated.

Thus far, I have focused on the economic dimensions of privatization, defined in terms of profit goals. Of equal importance are the *social development* purposes of human service systems. These have to do largely with morality and social responsibility and with necessarily rising costs of living in postagrarian (now postmodern?) societies. Social development is also concerned with the relationship between individual development and the development of the species in the throes of a social epoch characterized by drastic change (in lifestyles, work style, interpersonal behavior standards, meanings and understanding, communication, travel, human values, ethnic relationships,[11] much of which is induced by "miraculous" biotechnical innovation. Human services, *as essential instruments for social development* in industrialized and postindustrialized societies, are in no way protected from the risks of a "free" market since these services ride on the outer edge of its peaks and troughs, particularly when they are a part of that market. Economic recessions and depressions have their first impact on "research and development" and "service" programs, as the last twenty years have amply demonstrated. A lag in or neglect of broad *social development* imperatives in a posttechnological society can easily result from permitting human service systems to be dependent upon vicissitudes of the market. Indeed, their elimination or reduction during an economic crisis tends to aggravate the crisis. Arthur Okun has put it quite specifically: "Profit goals are contrary to goals of social well-being of the society as a whole . . . To the extent that the system succeeds, it generates an efficient economy. but the pursuit of efficiency necessarily creates inequalities. And hence society faces a trade-off between equality and efficiency."[12] Inevitably, inequality in a democratic system eventually destroys efficiency when it leads to social instability.

Closely associated with social development has been the high value placed on altruism in American societies, as noted by Alexis DeTocqueville and Gunnar Myrdal and enthusiastically described by John Ehrenreich.[13] Richard Titmuss in his classic work *The Gift Relationship: From Human Blood to Social Policy*[14] emphasizes the importance of a sense of self-worth that is derived from the motivation for and acts of giving and helping. A supportive community pergola, which sustains nonprofit human service organizations—as well as publicly managed caring systems—is the institutional manifestation of both private and public dignity and self-worth. The sense of "giving through self and community" in direct human contact provides the moral essence to the quality of the helping process, a necessary ingredient in the relationship between the helper and the helped in civil societies.

VALUE-CRITICAL ANALYSIS

The changing interpretations of the meaning of "private" (referred to earlier in this chapter) are an example of the necessity for detailed and radical value-critical analysis in planning human services. Understanding human services in proper "detail" means specifically identifying the *human* impact of social policy. A "radical" evaluation challenges traditional assumptions regarding the purposes, methods, and goals of social policy or particular social policies. Value-critical procedures also force attention to the linguistic confusions that permeate the human sciences and, by derivation, the human service professions.[15] Confusions such as these are widespread as they are inevitable, in part due to etymological processes of at least 300 years, which have been inordinately influenced by the language of mathematics and the natural, physical, and social sciences. Michel Foucault's penetrating work. *The Order of Things: An Archaeology of the Human Sciences* is especially informative on this issue.[16] Foucault argues that modern language developed effectively as an instrument to serve the natural and physical sciences; its form and use fits these disciplines better than the human science disciplines.

Some Assumptions

At least four principle assumptions represent categories of issues that demand attention in a much needed value-critical assessment of privatization for the future. These are the following:

- a global perspective on social policy (as compared to a national perspective);
- the fallacy of economic scarcity;
- the social polity and the market economy as related, *but separate*, institutions that govern American life; and
- new ways of knowing, or the significance of epistemological and etymological influences on the human sciences and the human services professions.[17]

The Global Perspective on Social Policy

National social policies can no longer be assessed without consideration of both international and worldwide implications. Advanced technology in cybernetics and transportation has sharpened our perception of the planet as a global community. Worldwide news is instantaneous and can be received at almost any point on the globe. "Virtual reality" can now be experienced literally; the international exchange of information is often instantaneous; technology and skills ride on the sound waves and light waves of modern communication and jet-thrusted travel. The transmission of scenes as well as sounds simultaneously confirms reality and encourages the dramatic dimension of communication. These technological elements have created societies in which members are protected against many of the social risks often precipitated by science and technology. However, four-fifths of the world's population is not protected.[18] In developed social systems, technology, human services, and entitlements need to operate hand in hand. ("High-tech" means "high touch," according to John Naisbett.)[19] While the provision of social entitlements and services to populations who are experiencing the frictional and structural changes generated by expanding technology are essential for stabilized, rational, civil, or "caring" social systems as well as for economic development, these policies have often been assigned lower priority to "economic" development, in spite of their necessity to achieve *economic development* in today's world.

We are, finally, beginning to notice the relations between national social policies and worldwide social policies. The phenomena of institutionalized human service systems, the rapid emergence of nations striving toward and achieving technical and social development, and mobile populations increasing in size and character are forces that impel consideration of international standards for levels of living and social relationships, as well as economic success. Can we envision world *social policy* dependent on the vicissitudes of international market systems, knowing that these operate with minimal regulation while they often promote outrageous human exploitation?[20]

Economic Scarcity

Economic scarcity is the basic rationale underlying market-driven, capitalist economies. Although classical economics and many contemporary economists assert the population of the world is not able to support its own growth, this assumption is probably inaccurate, despite the Report of the Club of Rome (1972) and other experts who deny that technological capacities will enable the maintenance of a resoundingly expanded world population. Recent reports released by the U.S. Department of Agriculture are more optimistic.[21] It seems clear now that the shortage of the food supply compared to population growth is based upon certain rarely acknowledged presumptions, such as the continuation of *unequal distribution* of food and other resources, both nationally and internationally. If unequal distribution between developed countries and underdeveloped countries, white races and nonwhite races, upper-class and lower-class populations, and the rich and the poor continues, the elimination of acute malnutrition and mass death by starvation will not be achieved. As low aggregate productivity is overcome by technological improvements and general socioeconomic development and as initiatives toward more accommodating relationships between nations and among peoples multiply, distribution problems can be expected to be reduced and social development to proceed balanced with population growth. World food prices have declined to historic lows, resulting from productivity improvements, and there is currently a worldwide surplus of grain. Total food production continues to grow much faster than the population (by 5 percent annually during the 1980s). The world has not reached, nor is it near, the upper limits of production capacity, according to many experts.[22]

Economic theories of scarcity are now subject to serious question. The growth potential as a result of technology has to be investigated more deeply and widely—the methodological approaches to human science research and the significance of new heuristic social-planning paradigms are examples of new-age thinking.[23] Improved future education of social policy experts and the importance of an international orientation in social policy are necessary requirements. With vigilant international surveillance, however, world trade can be restrained in its tendency to invite excessive windfall profits for expanded multinational business conglomerations, which most of the people of the world cannot afford. The principle of worldwide scarcity as a basic assumption for economics, if finally rejected, should have an important impact on the direction of social policy.

The Polity and the Market Economy

Political and social institutions (schools, governments, constitutions, courts) provide and ensure rights and privileges that eventually produce political and social equality. On the other hand, economic institutions rely on market-determined factors that generate disparities in living standards. Differentials in living standards result from an intolerably wide range of income levels, which tend to serve either as rewards or penalties. As such they seek to promote maximum efficiency in the use of resources, human and otherwise. The striking mixture of equal human and political rights and strikingly unequal economic opportunity precipitates tensions between the principles of democratic governments and the principles of free-market institutions. The economic system is much less structured, organized, and controlled than the political system, and as a result, it offers enormous risks and few protections for most. Human services are also exposed to these risks when they are subject to market freedom. While the market serves as an efficient system for spurring and channeling productive economic effort and for promoting experimentation and innovation, the protection of individual freedom of expression and opportunity has, too often, become subjected to the "tyranny of the dollar yardstick."[24]

New Ways of Knowing

While we have generated and accumulated knowledge and technology beyond the most optimistic expectations of its forebears, our species has not begun to realize the kinds of dramatic, radical, new orientations to obtaining knowledge that are required to create and maintain a stabilized and rational social system, either national or global.[25] Investigations of complex questions regarding methods of delivery of human services are hampered by epistemological systems that are "analytic" and "linear"[26] and fall short of the proper critical, heuristic, or phenomenological power necessary to deal with human interpersonal issues as contrasted, for example, with physical or mathematical issues. We have not discovered a theoretical base for the knowledge necessary for working with human interpersonal relationships in unique bureaucratic settings, such as human service organizations with rehabilitative, curative, or preventative social goals rather than profits. The character, structure, leadership, and management needs of human service organizations are not the same as those for organizations that build automobiles or manufacture shovels. Management systems in the profit sector are critically different from those systems in the human services sector. Some of these distinctions are well-known and self-evident. Some remain not articulated or yet to be discovered.

Martin Rein has argued that conventional analytic thinking is not sufficiently liberated to permit the kind of drastic radical "challenge," if you will, to conventional academic modes of investigation and expression in social policy. It is not adequate because philosophic and academic canons superimpose certain categories of knowledge and analysis that do not fit recently developed experiences in the social and human interpersonal spheres. Rein is influenced by Foucault's treatment of etymology in the human sciences and the resulting epistemological limitations. With value-critical analysis, Rein assumes an intellectual posture that challenges the basic premises of conventional beliefs regarding the value of the scientific method for many (not all) aspects of social policy. Okun's principle of the inverse relationship between equality and efficiency, for example, is challengable from the value perspective. Rein argues against cost-benefit (efficient) approaches for policy issues. He appears not so much concerned with values and morals for their own sake, but with the *futility* of attempting economic efficiency in matters of social policy.

It is of much more than passing interest that the group of theoretical constructs that Rein and other contemporary social science scholars find to be helpful in pursuing these questions are similarly applicable to direct social work practice as they are to social policy. This, however, is a subject for much more exploration elsewhere.[27]

SUMMARY AND CONCLUSIONS

The flight into the privatization of human service seems to result from a combination of select macro and micro social forces and human events during the past 20 or 25 years. As the largely mechanical intellectual methods of science and mathematics have enabled the conquest of nature, it was expected that human interpersonal, social, and community problems would respond similarly. This has not occurred.

With the sweep of conservative ideologies throughout the world, the exploitation of underdeveloped countries and countries in the process of their development continues from within as well as from the outside. However, as these new nations achieve advanced technological capacities, they increasingly seek to establish necessary

human support systems. The development process in human relations among populations and national states becomes strained and
suggests the new importance of global social policy. The sale of
human services for profit (privatization), therefore, becomes a
global issue, particularly in the context of powerful multinational
corporate growth.

From a pragmatic point of view, it is unlikely that the private
profit sector in the future will be interested in acquiring all helping
systems. From a moral point of view, the importance of volunteer-
ism in human service delivery systems cannot be overstated. Rein
has suggested that one way to deal with this is to abandon the
efficiency orientation in social policy for a value-critical orientation.
As an example, social workers true to their democratic-humanistic
traditions might yet attach themselves professionally to grassroots
movements and, from a scholarly perspective, to a value-critical
heuristic thinking mode in order to challenge the current premises of
Western social thought, which have brought us to this intellectual/
social impasse.

Thomas Kuhn's[28] theory of the paradigm shift might *conceivably*
apply to the present process of change in human service delivery
systems (from a welfare state model to a privatization model). A
paradigm shift is in order, but perhaps have we been looking at the
wrong paradigm as a replacement. The problem of the failure of the
welfare state is not so much a normal market phenomenon, as it has
been conventionally described, but is primarily a result of misap-
plication of methods of inquiry and scholarship that do not fit current social policy dilemmas. The shift that deserves the attention of
the human sciences and professions is the shift in *ways of knowing*,
a shift from the scientific paradigm (in pursuit of truth) to what has
been identified as the "heuristic paradigm"[29] (in pursuit of discovery). Scholars in the human sciences and in social work have
recently been uncovering new concepts and models of investigation
of knowledge that suggest an epistemological paradigm shift for the
social sciences and (by derivation) for the human service professions will occur. The work of Martin Rein on value-critical thinking
and more recently that of Pieper, Tyson, Weik, Laird, and Hartman[30]
on heuristic approaches to knowing, among others, point out that
our problem in designing systems for delivering social services has

less to do with the structure of services or society or economic theory as we understand them than with our perception of a rational society. Our processes for planning and designing institutionalized human services, rather than relying on a system that presumes an economics of scarcity, should explore heuristic means of investigation of the human condition from a *value-critical perspective*.

NOTES

1. Rein, 1983, p. ix.
2. Ibid.
3. For a respectable model of the welfare state, see Morris, 1974.
4. Drucker, 1993, p. 120.
5. Titmuss, 1959.
6. See, for example Reid and Popple (eds.), 1992; and Galbraith, 1992.
7. See de Schweinitz, 1947; also Francis and Sherman, in Griffiths (ed.), 1994, pp. 40-41.
8. See Gilder, 1981.
9. Nelson, 1992, pp. 815-828.
10. Ibid.
11. Gitlin, 1989, p. 100.
12. Okun, 1975, p. 1.
13. DeTocqueville, 1993; Myrdal, 1962; Ehrenreich, 1985.
14. Titmuss, 1971.
15. See Lorraine, 1996, p. 119.
16. Foucault, 1989. See Chapter 5 especially.
17. See for example, Foucault, 1989; Polkinghorne, 1983; Rein, 1983; Roberts, 1990; Tyson, 1992, pp. 541-556; Pieper, 1989, pp. 8-34; Ehrenreich, 1985.
18. *United Nations,* June 1996.
19. aisbett, 1982.
20. Griffiths, 1994, pp. 32-94; Barry, 1987, pp. 21-66.
21. Budiansky, 1994, pp. 58-59.
22. Rabenson, 1994, pp. 58-59.
23. Hassard and Parker, 1993, p. 8.
24. Okun, p. 119.
25. Hartman, 1990, pp. 3-4.
26. Lorraine, 1996, p. 119.
27. Vigilante, 1994.
28. Kuhn, 1970.
29. See Tyson, 1995.
30. Hartman, 1990; Laird, in Vigilante and Lewis (eds.), 1993; Pieper, 1989; Tyson, 1992.

BIBLIOGRAPHY

Barry, Tom. *Roots of Rebellion: Land & Hunger in Central America*. Boston, MA: South End Press, 1987.

Budiansky, Stephen. "10 Billion for Dinner, Please." *U.S. News and World Report*, September 12, 1994.

DeLuca, Burton C. Letter to the Editor. *The New York Times*, August 26, 1994.

DeSchweinitz, Karl. *England's Road to Social Security*. Philadelphia, PA: University of Pennsylvania Press, 1947.

DeTocqueville, Alexis. *Democracy in America*. New York: Alfred A. Knopf, 1993.

Drucker, Peter. *Post Capitalist Society*. New York: HarperCollins Publications, 1993.

Ehrenreich, John. *The Altruistic Imagination*. Ithaca, NY: Cornell University Press, 1985.

Foucault, Michel. *The Order of Things: An Archaeology of the Human Sciences*. New York: The Free Press, 1989.

Francis, Michael J., and Amy Sherman. "Rethinking Development: A Market Friendly Strategy for the Poor." In Robert J. Griffiths (ed.), *Annual Edition Third World 94/95*. The Dushkin Publishing Group, Inc., Sluice Dock, CN: Guilford Press, 1994, pp. 40-41.

Galbraith, John Kenneth. *The Culture of Contentment*. New York: Houghton Mifflin Co., 1992.

Gilder, George. *Wealth and Poverty*. New York: Basic Books, 1981.

Gitlin, Todd. "Postmodernism: Roots and Politics, What Are They Talking About?" *Dissent*, Winter, 1989, p. 100.

Griffiths, Robert J. (ed.) *Annual Editions Third World 94/95*. The Dushkin Publishing Group, 1994.

Hartman, Ann. "Many Ways of Knowing." *Social Work*, 35, 1-96, January 1990.

Hassard, John, and Martin Parker (eds.). *Postmodernism and Organizations*. Newbury Park, CA: Sage Publications, 1993.

Kuhn, Thomas. *The Structure of Scientific Revolutions*, second edition. International Encyclopedia of Unified Science, Foundations of the Unity of Science, Chicago: University of Chicago Press, 1970.

Laird, Joan. "Revisioning Social Work Education." In Florence Vigilante and Harold Lewis (eds.), *Journal of Teaching in Social Work*, 8 (1/2), 1993.

Lorraine, Tamsin. Bill Martin, *Matrix and Line: Derrida and the Possibilities of Postmodern Social Theory, Journal of Philosophy and Social Criticism*, 3, 1996, p. 119.

Morris, Robert. *Toward A Caring Society*. Columbia University: School of Social Work, 1974.

Myrdal, Gunnar. *An American Dilemma: The Negro Problem and Modern Democracy*. New York: Harper and Row Publishers, 1962.

Naisbett, John. *Megatrends: Ten New Directions Transforming Our Lives*. New York: Warner Books, 1982.

Nelson, J. "Social Welfare and the Market Economy." *Social Science Quarterly*, 73 (4), 1992.

Okun, Arthur. *Equality and Efficiency: The Big Tradeoff.* Washington, DC: The Brookings Institution, 1975.

Pieper, Martha Heineman. "The Heuristic Paradigm: A Unifying and Comprehensive Approach to Social Work Research." *Smith College Studies in Social Work*, 60 (1), November 1989.

Polkinghorne, Donald. *Methodology for the Human Sciences: Systems of Inquiry.* Albany: State University of New York Press, 1983.

Rabenson, B. H. "U.S. Department of Agriculture Research Services." *U.S. News and World Report*, September 12, 1994.

Reid, P. Nelson, and Philip R. Popple. *The Moral Purposes of Social Work: The Character and Intentions of a Profession.* Chicago, IL: Nelson Hall Publishers, 1992.

Rein, Martin. *From Policy to Practice.* Armonk, NY: M. E. Sharpe, Inc., 1983.

Roberts, Richard. *Lessons from the Past: Issues for Social Work Theory.* New York: Tavistock/Routledge, 1990.

Stoesz, D. "Corporate Welfare." *Social Work*, 31, 1986.

Titmuss, Richard. *Essays on "The Welfare State."* New Haven, CT: Yale University Press, 1959.

Titmuss, Richard. *The Gift Relationship: From Human Blood to Social Policy*, New York: Pantheon Books, 1971.

Tyson, Katherine B. "A New Approach to Relevant Scientific Research for Practitioners: The Heuristic Paradigm." *Social Work*, 37 (6), 1992.

Tyson, Katherine B. *New Foundations for Scientific Social and Behavioral Research: The Heuristic Paradigm.* Needham, MA: Allyn and Bacon, 1995.

Vigilante, J. L. *"The Moral Purposes of Social Work: The Character and Intentions of A Profession,"* (Book Review). *Journal of Teaching in Social Work*, 9 (1/2), 1994.

Chapter 8

Legal Regulation and Accreditation: Obstacles to Practice

Juan Ramos

Although social work practice and the profession as a whole has consistently identified with and utilized general systems theory as it applies to interpersonal relationships, it is important to note that the infrastructure of the social work profession is indeed itself a system that often represents rigidity and a system in which change is difficult as it is in many other aspects of social living. This analysis will attempt to identify some of the forces that are at work in considering the issues inherent in legal regulation and accreditation in social work education. It will also address the potentials for change. We can start with the assumption that the profession of social work has an ongoing interest in and commitment to social change, yet often change is hard to achieve and difficult to experience. The question to be raised at this time when the institution of social welfare and the social work profession is facing serious obstacles in performing their respective missions is, how can the infrastructure of the profession be sensitized to the need for self analysis and change? An additional critical need for the profession, at this point in its history, is to seriously engage in effective research to validate its body of knowledge and to create new tested knowledge.

TRIANGULAR MODELS OF RELATIONSHIPS

A helpful mechanism for conceptualizing such issues is the concept of triangular relationships. One side of the triangle represents the public, the legislators who represent them, and those who are service consumers. The second side of the triangle is the leadership of organized profession while the third side consists of the member-ship of the organized profession. The latter, generally, represents the force that could energize the process of interaction between all three sides.

Change in the profession's policy toward legal regulation is diffi-cult at this point to consider since currently there is no organized constituency that seems to be willing to invest time, energy, and resources in engaging in active participation for change. Most mem-bers of the profession, generally, support the concept of legal regula-tion, although there may be some small differences in where they think the emphasis should be placed. However, unless an organized constituency can emerge with a serious challenge, it is questionable that there can be a significant debate. When a constituency cares deeply enough about a social problem, becomes organized, and is willing to invest energy to engage in a struggle to solve the problem, the critical segment of this triangle can be activated. The second segment of the triangle becomes energized when an organization or public policy making group becomes involved. The third segment is created when the public agency or other entities that have jurisdic-tion over services that can address the problem become involved.

Another conceptual triangle for consideration exists in relation-ship to the profession of social work. These legs are (1) research, (2) education, and (3) practice. Research informs education and education informs both research and practice. This triangular rela-tionship for the social work profession, currently, does not seem to be operating effectively. Social work colleagues at the National Institute of Mental Health are fond of calling this triangle "the three-legged stool," but with a warning not to sit on it since one of the legs is extremely weak, the leg called research. Without the strong leg of research, the dynamic interaction necessary to energize this critical interaction leading to professional competence cannot be successfully developed. This triangle has a significant impact on accreditation, licensing, and certification, as well as on social work and social work education. Other forces that also impact this triangle are the implications of Title VI, of the Civil Rights Act of 1964. A third triangle is the one that produces policy formulation. One leg is power or influence, the second is values or ideology, and the third leg is science, namely the utilization of knowledge that comes from competent research findings. This latter triangle can assist us in appreciating the domestic policymaking process that is so important to the social work profession. It is especially helpful in understanding the important role of organized constituent groups.

CRISES IN THE FIELD OF SOCIAL WORK

The mid- and late-1990s present a series of crises that challenge the near future of the social work profession. For a number of years, this profession has had a significant opportunity to define itself anew to the U.S. public. This was especially true after the fall of the Soviet Union and the removal of the threat of socialism to the American free-enterprise system. Throughout its history, social workers were seen as associated with the value of collectivism, the economic ideology of socialism, and occasionally, the political ideology of communism. The social policy stance of the National Association of Social Workers, which nationally and locally supported income redistribution programs and remained committed to the poor and other oppressed populations gave some support to those who were critical of this professions "leftist" leanings. Social work's fundamental value orientations are surely not calculated to find favor in America's main stream capitalist, free-market environment. The profession is also committed to such liberal social policies as affirmative action, federal legal entitlements to a number of social benefits, and an increasing social welfare state. With the demise of the Soviet Union, the external threat of communism and socialism to the American political and economic systems has significantly receded. This should have presented a unique opportunity to clarify what the social work profession advocates.

A recent example of how social work was misunderstood and maligned was the national debate over the crime bill, which was described in the media as a "sock-work pork-piece of legislation." Social work services, which were included in the bill for the purposes of crime prevention, were termed "social pork." The critical comment was "if you called 911 for a law enforcement officer, you did not want to get a social worker." The Heritage Foundation described the crime bill as providing for too few police officers and too many social workers.

There is now, and there will continue to be, a major national debate about the social problem of a financing medical care costs. Although related, medical care can be separated from health care and from public health. Most of the health resources and national attention is currently going to medical care, and there is grave concern for continuously escalating costs. When special attention to health care financing reform was projected by President Clinton, little focus was placed on the area of public health. Excluded from the debate were issues of prevention addressing such items as diet, exercise, and smoking, as well as other risk factors usually associated with poor health. The key issue in illness prevention and public health is the crucial connection between health and behavior. Because of their behavioral expertise, social workers in health care can make a significant contribution to public health. They can and do contribute heavily to medical care, but their major contribution is, and should be, to public health. The health professions including social work are in good a position to move public health significantly forward at this time. This connection has not yet been fully developed. The opportunity currently exists to expand the social work role in health care if the profession moves in a direction of greater involvement in public health. Because medical care has high public acceptance, there has been a tendency to medicalize social issues and social problems and to put these issues and problems under the medical aegis. Medical care, therefore, has garnered more resources on the basis that this approach is the most effective one.

HOMELESSNESS, HIV/AIDS, AND VIOLENCE

Three major social problems in the last several years have highlighted the need for a definition that is broader than that of "medical." The three that have raised concerns about the validity of the medical care approach to social problems are: homelessness, HIV/AIDS, and violence. In all three instances, there have been major efforts to medicalize these issues. This has been accepted by the nonmedical professions, including social work, because there seem to be more resources in the medical area and there appears to be greater promise of success within the medical reference. The publicly funded programs of Medicaid and Medicare also provide considerable resources to finance medical care programs. The three aforementioned social problems must, however, be addressed from a public health perspective in order for effective solutions to be developed. The social work role within public health has great potential to contribute to effective resolutions to the problems of homelessness, violence, and HIV/AIDS and also to enhance the recognition of social work. This profession has been blocked from defining its role or claiming the state in these areas because of the lack of proactive leadership at the national level. There has been little attempt to stake the claim of social work in providing solutions to these problems. There is a need to raise voices that can provide clarity as to how the social work profession can effectively address these problems. A 1993 issue of the *New England Journal of Medicine* highlights this perspective boldly. The author makes the case for a social policy for health and strongly advocates for a national institute of social health as a way of addressing public health and health care as separate from medical care.

MANAGED HEALTH CARE

Another current issue relates to managed behavioral health care. There has been resistance by some members of the social work profession to embrace case management as a legitimate social work function. Many social workers are currently called "case managers." This term is one that originates from the world of business. It seems to reflect a mainstream positive quality and brings with it a high degree of acceptability and potential support from the business sector. It utilizes such management concepts as cost-effectiveness, cost efficiency, effective productivity, and success in achieving goals. There are rapid developments at many state levels in the area of managed behavioral health care. A number of states are turning their Medicaid funds over to private for-profit contractors. Some states have been doing this for many years. Arizona contracts all of its mental health federal block-grant funds and its allocated state funds to a private contractor, who then in turn subcontracts with individual providers. The states of Massachusetts and Wisconsin have also moved in this direction. Hawaii has been involved in such a program for several years. There is a sense that this process can reduce or contain costs. There are concerns from some providers, but the payers, most often insurance companies, seem to be very pleased with the profits that are generated. Managed behavioral health care has as its goal cost-effectiveness. However, the issue of public funds being used by private, for-profit firms must raise some deep concerns for the social work profession. The bottom-line question is the validity of such contracts for the welfare of the service's consumer.

The state of California, for the first time, has established cultural and linguistic requirements in managed care. Contractors must now operationalize these requirements. Since a large portion of the eligible population in the state of California is comprised of members of minority groups, the question has arisen concerning how effectively these contractors are providing services to this population.

Psychiatrists, and other clinicians in private practice, have been concerned over the years with cultural aspects of mental illness. The DSM-IV is now more appropriate for use in the multicultural society of this nation than ever before and also is appropriate for utilization in the global context to which it is being increasingly applied. The DSM-IV is now less biased to North American subcultural orientations and is more open to cross-cultural variations. It is also more practically useful and valid when applied to the context of diverse ethnic groups. Therefore, the DSM-IV can now function more validly as an international diagnostic system, which, in fact, it is now fast becoming in practice. The DSM-IV has two major parts that address ethnic and cultural considerations. One is contained in the introduction. The other part is in the appendix titled "Outline for Cultural Formulation and Glossary of Culture Bound Syndromes."

A committee headed by Dr. Juan Mezzich from the University of Pittsburgh has made a major contribution to the new DSM-IV by including three types of information specially related to cultural considerations:

1. A discussion in the text of cultural variations in the clinical presentations of those disorders that have been included in the classification;

2. A description of cultural-bound syndromes that have not been included in the classifications (these are included in the appendix); and
3. An outline for cultural formulation designed to assist the clinician in systematically evaluating and reporting the impact of the individual's cultural context.

ACCREDITATION, LICENSING, AND CERTIFICATION

In considering the issue of legal regulation for the social work profession, cultural considerations become relevant to three terms: accreditation, licensing, and certification.

The term "accredit" means to consider or recognize as outstanding, to give official authorization to, or approval of, to recognize or vouch for as confirming with a standard, or to recognize—like an educational institution maintains standards that qualify the graduates for admission to higher, or more specialized institutions, or for professional practice. All Masters of Social Work (MSW) programs in the United States are accredited by the Council on Social Work Education.

The term "certify" means to document, attesting that one has fulfilled the education or experience requirements in order to practice in the respective fields. It also means to attest as deemed through, or as represented by, meeting a particular standard.

"License" is permission to act, granted by a competent authority in order to engage in a business, occupation, or activity otherwise unlawful. It is a document evidencing a license granted to a person who has undergone training and obtained a license, as from a state conferring authorization to provide services. These definitions provide sanction and are the basis of the power implied in these three terms. They have been operationalized in many very powerful mechanisms and are directed essentially at protecting society from quacks and incompetents. A graduate from an accredited school of social work, therefore, with a state license or certification has sanction that what has been learned at school and what will be applied in practice will at the least not be harmful to societal members who may seek to use that particular service. Thus, a person with certification or licensing cannot be labeled as a quack or incompetent. However, serious questions can be raised and have been raised about the validity of the accreditation, licensing, and/or certification process. For example, there is a Council on Accreditation for Services for Families and Children, which is sponsored by six or seven national service organizations. This group claims that private accreditation is an especially American solution for the problem of assuring that agency providers of education, health care, or other social services meet the recognized standard of their domains and their professionals. The accreditation of the agency provider is part of a larger system of quality control and includes an accreditation of training programs and institutions as well as the certification and licensing of individual professionals. This council points out that it is an entity designed to protect society from organizations and persons who do not meet their standards.

The infrastructure of legal regulation and accreditation has been developed and established over a number of years and has become a very powerful mechanism. Since there is not yet an organized constituency willing to challenge this infrastructure mechanism, it has not become a public issue.

One of the original groups in the accreditation system was the Joint Commission on Accreditation of Healthcare Organizations. The Joint Commission was formed in 1951 as a private, not-for-profit organization to enhance the quality of health care provided to the public by establishing contemporary standards, evaluating health care organizations, rendering accreditation decisions, and providing education and consultative support to health care professions.

However, one can raise the question as to whether or not the Joint Commission utilizes cultural and linguistic requirements as criteria for accreditation in order to best serve ethnic and racial population groups. The Joint Commission, in fact, does not incorporate such cultural and linguistic requirements in their standards, and one should not expect an initiative in this direction unless some external groups make it an issue.

Another part of the infrastructure is the Health Care Financing Administration (HCFA), and within it, the Health Standards and Quality Bureau, which surveys and certifies medical records and staff for provider status. This includes private and public psychiatric hospitals and allows the certified providers to bill and be reimbursed by Medicaid and Medicare.

The third group, relevant to the accreditation process, is the Council on Recognition of Postsecondary Accreditation (CORPA). When this organization was first formed in 1975, it was known as COPA, the Council on Postsecondary Accreditation. For the first time, there was a national nongovernmental organization devoted exclusively to postsecondary accreditation. The accreditation informs the public that their accredited institution or program operates at an acceptable level of educational quality and integrity. CORPA recognizes national and regional institutional accredited bodies and specialized accredited bodies. The Council on Social Work Education, for instance, is recognized by CORPA as that specialized accrediting body for social work professional educational institutions. They also recognize bodies like the Mid-Atlantic Association of Colleges and Universities, as well as others that accredit colleges and universities in particular regions. The question to be posed to this group is the following: Are issues of diversity, multiculturalism, and racial and ethnic concerns incorporated into the criteria and standards for accreditation? Unfortunately, they do not exist in CORPA, but they do in some of the recognized bodies, such as the Council on Social Work Education.

Another organization to be considered is the Council on Accreditation for Families and Children. A similar question can be addressed to this group. The national and state examinations, such as those for the licensed or certified social workers, teachers, psychologists, etc., are the instruments by which legal regulation of practice takes place. An increasing number of service programs now require that staff be licensed or certified by the state in which they practice. Are there examination questions in the tests provided by this group that relate to work with clients or patients from other language or cultural groups?

Assessment or diagnostic instruments such as the DSM-IV are often required in most service programs and are often tied to reimbursement of services. For the most part, these instruments lack criteria relevant to language and cultural groups.

Finally, there are the board members and executive staff of the major national health, mental health, and human services organizations, which actively promote policies and whose members influence the appropriation of resources through their interaction with members of Congress. This part of the infrastructure system has considerable power over organizational service delivery, staffing, and the revaluation of services including diagnostic and treatment activities. In order to survive, agencies must meet the criteria of the accrediting, licensing, and certifying bodies. However, the board and staff members do not seem to be strong advocates for change even though it is apparent that there often is a mismatch between the criteria of accrediting bodies and the clients or patients who are being served.

What, therefore, are the consequences of the legal regulation policies and the accreditation bodies? Major segments of the American people seem to have given up on the socialization process, which includes the use of human services. They seem to feel that social services are often more harmful than productive. They question the necessity of many of the human services and wonder whether more problems are being created then are being solved, since poverty, crime, and violence continue to increase. Instead, many of the public seem to have opted for social control, i.e., more police, more prisons, and more resources for the criminal justice system. People seem to feel these days that control works and that it is effective. The answer seems to be to arrest as many violators as possible and to put them away for as long a period of time as possible. The negative consequence of such policies are never considered. The discussion, debate, and opinion to the recent federal crime bill clearly supports this observation. The three Ps—police, prisons, and prevention—probably made sense until the concept of prevention became somehow linked to social work and became labeled as "social pork" in its most negative connotation, implying wasteful and unnecessary misuse of taxpayers' money. The crime bill, when revisited by the Republican majority, will probably culminate in all of the funds in the prevention part being zeroed out and transferred to prisons and police. Prevention today has lost its credibility to the public. There no longer seems to be a belief that people can be socialized into the model of upstanding citizenship.

To what extent, therefore, are the current accreditation, certification, and licensing criteria and their related processees making it more difficult for social workers to provide quality services to people in need so that the human services can be restored to their importance in the socialization process? In other words, should the criteria for accrediting the educational programs of the helping professions be reviewed and revised? Will they be able to match the needs of the people who are to be served by these policies? Should the certification process also be overhauled to address the issues of cultural diversity? If not, social work will continue to lose whatever support still remains for the social services or for the continuation of the socialization process.

A great deal is at stake for the social welfare institution and the profession of social work. It is difficult, however, to project a positive scenario for the future. In any given year, there are about 100 national conferences and workshops on cultural competence, cultural sensitivity, cultural diversity, and people of color. Such conferences might be beneficial to professionals who are graduates of accredited schools. Should we continue to provide cultural sensitivity training and cultural diversity training for graduates or should something be done earlier and more efficiently as part of the formal educational process at the undergraduate and graduate level? All human service programs should require the accreditation standards to include a significant amount of cultural diversity content. In addition all state licensing and certification examinations should include questions related to work with culturally diverse populations. If a sizable number of people fail such an examination in that cultural area, it would then pose a major problem for the schools and result in a major change in the curriculum. Short of this, little change will take place.

Title VI of the Civil Rights Act of 1964 has recently observed its thirtieth anniversary. This law has been on the books, obviously, for a long time. The Department of Health and Human Services, however, has not yet developed regulations to implement Title VI. In 1978 and 1979, a major effort was undertaken to develop guidelines for such implementation but nothing came from this effort. A law firm in Washington, DC, took on the battle on behalf of a number of national racial and ethnic minority organizations for the development of such implementing regulations. This effort ended in 1981 when the talk about deregulation became strong. It, therefore, was impossible to push for the development of such regulations.

One contractor is currently assessing how racial and ethnic majorities are being serviced by the social services mental health organizations and health agencies at the local level. They will attempt to discover examples of where productive work is being done in this area and the way in which it works, as well as examples that do not seem to work well.

Title VI, in its implementing regulations, prohibits recipients of federal financial assistance from the Department of Health and Human Services from discriminating against persons based on race, color, or national origin. The regulation states that a recipient may not directly go through contractual or other arrangements, using criteria or methods of administration that have the effect of subjecting individuals to discrimination because of their race, color, or national origin. A recipient's failure to provide bilingual services to persons with limited English proficiency has, in certain circumstances, been held to have a discriminatory effect on such persons by depriving them of equal access to, and by limiting their participation in, the recipient's program. This is clearly in violation of Title VI.

The question before dedicated and committed social work professionals is how to develop strategies to restore the image of the profession by reassessing and revising the concept of social work's function in this society. This profession needs to do more than merely pick up the pieces created by the negative impact of our capitalist economic system upon oppressed citizens in our society. Harry Specht and Mark Courney's book *Unfaithful Angels: How Social Work Has Abandoned Its Mission* (1995, by the Free Press) documents how professional social workers seem to have abandoned the public sector in child welfare, income maintenance, and mental health among others. What is the current image of the social work profession to the public? This is the time for leadership of the profession to develop a major strategy to raise the hard questions and put to the test some of the classic assumptions of the profession. National leadership is desperately needed to move the profession toward utilization of research-based knowledge.

RESEARCH

Great strides have been made by the nursing profession in its research agenda. A decision was made by nursing professional leaders that research would have to become an important part of the profession. They mobilized themselves and acted upon it. Today, within the National Institutes of Health, there is a National Institute on Nursing Research with a budget of fifty-two million dollars. They also receive research money from NIMH (National Institute of Mental Health). Today, in many hospitals and other medical settings, nurses are replacing social workers in a number of functions that historically social workers have claimed as their turf. In terms of scientific research, social work may be twenty years behind the times. There seems to be, within the social work profession, an antiscience, anti-intellectual, and antiresearch sentiment. The profession is seen by professionals primarily as service deliverers, and many social workers feel that the profession has no business conducting research. Yet about 70 percent of the mental health workforce are social workers. How valid is the knowledge base that social workers utilize to formulate their interventions? Effective mental health intervention needs more than an art form; it needs a science base.

Recently, five national social work organizations contributed funds to develop the Institute for the Advancement of Social Work Research. This represents a major message to the profession as well as to other helping professions. The congressional appropriation committees have very positive messages about the need for social work research. In the appropriations language pertaining to the National Cancer Institute, the National Heart, Lung, and Blood Institute, and others, reference is made that social workers were beginning to play an important part, in social support, for persons with cancer and that research funds should be provided in order to document the effect of these interventions. The language directed the National Cancer Institute, for instance, to provide research funds to social workers for this purpose.

The number of people applying to schools of social work seems to be increasing significantly. These applicants are for the most part dedicated and committed people. They must have a curriculum that is supported by framework and infrastructure that has accreditation standards and licensing criteria that will prepare them adequately for the reality of diversity and for the priority of service to the oppressed populations in society.

Only then can graduates or professional social work education programs have a fighting chance to making a significant difference and to help raise the profession to a place where it can accomplish its maximum potential.

Chapter 9

Challenges of Managed Care for Health Professionals: Implications for Social Work Practice

Gary Rosenberg

Of all the issues that impinge upon the current health care scene, affecting both consumers and providers, managed care presents the greatest challenge. This phenomenon is already giving ample evidence of its impact upon the entire health care system and contains major critical implications for social work practice in the health care arena.

The health care system today is a rapidly changing one; the subsystems are now beginning to merge into larger units. The structure of finance and service delivery is changing rapidly as well. Managed care as a method of financing and service delivery is making a dramatic impact on the organization of the health care system. Using what are called "penetration rates," we can analyze how much managed-care activity exists in any particular marketplace and what effect it has on that marketplace. There is a trend to blur roles between providers and consumers so that insurance companies, including the not-for-profit ones such as Blue Cross/Blue Shield of New Jersey have not purchased primary care networks of physicians. Insurance companies now employ physicians. The traditional distinctions between those who pay for and those who provide no longer exist, particularly, in the more mature managed-care marketplaces. Competition is accelerating if one looks at the advertising budgets of various health centers when one can learn a great deal about competition in health care. There seems little question that there will continue to be a shrinkage of organizations in the health care system. A small number of corporate groups will emerge as controlling and dominating the health care system in the United States in the near future.

The paradigms, in health care, are also changing. In the 1960s, the marketplace consisted of individual providers. In the 1980s, there began to merge some networking activity. By the year 2000, there will be "unmanaged competition" rather than "managed competition" except, perhaps, in a state like New York and five or six others. Health insurance, in the 1960s, was indemnity insurance. In the 1980s, there emerged indemnity insurance mixed with HMOs and PPOs (Preferred Provider Organizations). In the year 2000, there will be a market of at least 50 percent in managed care and perhaps more. Reimbursement, in the 1960s, was charged a base and it was per diem; therefore, it paid to keep patients in the hospital. Hospitals became the cash cow of health care. In the 1980s, there was a move from retrospective reimbursement to prospective reimbursement using a system called DRGs (Diagnostic-Related Groups). In the service of cost containment, the DRG identified an average length of hospital stay and a set amount of reimbursement. In the year 2000 as even today, we will see capitation as a form of financing involving risk taking on the part of physicians and hospitals. There will be direct contracting between insurers and providers. In the 1960s, the core provider was the hospital, which then became a medical center. Hospitals in the future will no longer be the core of the health care system. One of the problems for social workers, in this future scenario, is that the hospital, where most social workers are now employed, will no longer offer the same employment opportunities. This poses a dilemma. How can the social work profession in health care move from the hospital to where the action will be in the future, mainly in the community, the primary care offices, and the ambulatory care settings? That is where social workers in health care will have to move. The main funding for health, however, will come through capitation. Capitated care will prohibit the use of the hospital except when absolutely necessary. It will limit expensive procedures for diagnosis and laboratory tests. There are sure to be some deficiencies in this type of managed care although it may help to make more appropriate use of resources. Today, it could be effectively argued that such efficiencies are not taking place.

The history of hospitals in this country reflects the fact that they were built by their local communities, unlike in Europe, where hospitals were largely built by universities. In the United States, a community-built hospital was in a contract with its community to take care of its health needs. Community service standards and community benefits standards were frequently argued. In the 1980s, the tertiary care hospitals sought to expand their geographical regions. Today, the problem is how to identify the responsibility of health care toward the local community. Unless people have local access to health care, how can they relate to the health system? Hospitals no longer look to their local communities in the way that they did before. That poses an additional dilemma.

The care components for inpatient services, in the 1960s, emphasized maximum utilization of the hospital inpatient and outpatient services. Today, we can design a full continuum of care from prevention and health promotion all the way through tertiary care, but little of it takes place within the hospital. Physicians, in the 1960s, were in solo practice and they seemed to enjoy it. They were independent and self-directed practitioners. In the 1980s, there was a movement toward group practice and group specialization. The number of physicians in the United States increased 190 percent between 1960 and 1990. Primary care practice, however, only increased 15 percent. There was an overproduction of specialists and administrative physicians. In the year 2000, we will see employed physicians and a rising demand for primary care. These were the developments that brought managed care to the fore.

Rhonda Cuttlechuck, of New York City, a health care specialist and advocate, claims that health care in New York City is "a spectrum of help with a system out of balance." What makes this system out of balance is that most of the resources now go to acute care, the hospitals. Fewer resources go to the laboratory, to prevention, to public health, and to primary care. Even less go to supportive care housing, home health care, hospice, respite care, and for the support of people in their own environments.

Hopefully, what will emerge is a system in balance, with health education, health promotion, and health status of communities becoming important areas. Primary care also needs to return to its former importance. Acute care and tertiary hospitals will diminish in both their acquisition of resources and their utilization of resources. For the booming aging population, nursing homes, rehabilitation facilities, assisted living, and home support programs are the places where the health care dollars, and the social services dollars should be directed. This then represents a system much more in balance, one which, hopefully, will be the future direction.

Health care costs as a percentage of gross national product are expected to rise to 17 percent and to exceed a trillion dollars by the year 2000. The increase in the cost of medical care insurance for the U.S. corporate sector as part of companies' benefit structure rose approximately 70 percent since 1960. Corporations have been extremely concerned about the issue of medical insurance cost containment. This factor has made the issue a relevant one both nationally and in the individual states. National health insurance, however, is not in the forecast for this nation in the near future. No major national social policy, with the exception of the Social Security Act of 1935, has been approved in the United States until at least 50 percent of the states have implemented it in some form in their own state laws. In the health insurance arena, we are nowhere close to that percentage today. The social focus for action I suggest should be the state governments. That is where the National Association of Social Workers (NASW) and other health insurance advocates need to look for change to take place.

What effect did this fiscal explosion have on the health care industry? Hospital admissions in the United States rose to a high point in 1981 and 1982. There were 36.4 million admissions in 1982. By 1989 this number was down to 31.1 million admissions. Was this because people were healthier? No! Another 70 percent loss by the year 2000 is expected so that inpatient numbers will shrink to about 25 million, down from the high point of 36 million in 1982. Considering the demographics of a growing aging population, a Medicare population, and an expanding general population, this drop poses an interesting question. Simultaneously, ambulatory care health services have increased 40 percent between 1985 and 1989. By the year 2000, this will increase another 106 percent to about 450 million outpatient visits.

Social workers thinking about job placements in health care should no longer focus on working in the inpatient hospital system, but rather working in the community and in ambulatory care, as well as in primary care. What roles, however, can social workers play in health prevention and promotion? How can the vulnerable, in our society, be identified? How can social workers get paid for what they do in these areas? Outpatient revenue has gone up significantly since 1985 as have prices. It is not only a result of increased volume, but the rising prices of services, which have produced greater revenues. The result is that ambulatory care revenues have now reached about 25 percent of the total revenue of health care organizations, which includes both hospitals and ambulatory care facilities.

These then are some of the facts that bring us to the issue of managed care. Managed care has been promulgated by liberals and conservatives both, as a method to achieve one goal, namely, cost-effective, cost-efficient health care delivery. It attracts a strange group of bedfellows. It is used to characterize a wide range of health plans from indemnity insurance through HMOs and fully capitated plans. The definition of managed care includes any plan that incorporates mechanisms to monitor and authorize the use of health services.

An indemnity plan may require a second opinion for surgery or preauthorization. Managed care actually began in indemnity insurance. It also incorporates negotiated payment methods and utilization controls dealing with both price and volume.

Managed care is not synonymous with access since it does not guarantee access to health care. Some believe that even with a managed-care plan, one may not have full access to health care. Many managed-care plans, particularly those within the for-profit companies, use the denial process for marketing. Managed Medicaid is another, fairly new development. The goal for New York State is to have 50 percent of Medicaid recipients enrolled in a managed care plan within the next five-year period. The experience in East Harlem is an interesting example of great liberties in marketing. When people in East Harlem were enrolled in a plan, they were told that they could use the Mt. Sinai Hospital, and of course, they could keep the same physician that they had before. This, however, has not proven to be true. In fact, once people enrolled in a managed-care plan, they were then disenrolled from Medicaid and then reenrolled in a plan that does not necessarily use their former physician, or other services for their hospital of choice. Another example of what we may call the "managed-care denial game," is that rules and regulations are then promulgated, which have the effect of obstructing people's use of service. For instance, if a patient does not receive a preauthorization, and receives five or six sessions of treatment before discovering that such preauthorization was necessary, then the provider is usually not reimbursed. Managed-care companies, particularly the for-profit organizations, earn anywhere from 20 to 30 percent in profit, which represents a significant addition to health care costs.

There are three mechanisms used by managed-care companies to contain costs and maximize their profits. One is the denial of free choice of doctor and/or hospital. The company substitutes lower-cost providers. They may not be of lower quality, but they are lower in cost and are willing to follow the managed-care guidelines. They generally negotiate on the protocols used by the managed-care companies and they negotiate on price. Usually, the price is somewhat less than what providers normally charge. The managed-care companies also erect rigid barriers to access. It does not seem to matter whether one uses the system a great deal or a little; the barriers still exist. The third mechanism to contain costs is micromanagement by what is termed "invisible diagnosticians." These people—some are social workers—are employed by insurance companies and are empowered by them to make the decision about the course of treatment based upon protocols, which are reliable in that they are, consistently, followed. These protocols may not necessarily be valid ones. These protocols do not suggest that the treatment recommended is necessarily the best available. No one seems to know to whom these "invisible diagnosticians" are accountable. It is very difficult to track professional accountability in this arena of managed care.

The popular culture concern is reflected in a Doonesbury cartoon, which comments on managed care. A doctor is explaining to the insurance representative what he plans to do in the way of treatment. The insurance representative says, "That's overkill, why not just do an X ray?" In the next panel the insurance representative proceeds to actually perform the surgery. Everyone connected with medical care seems to be concerned about this important issue of "micromanagement."

Managed care, as a system, is currently evolving and, obviously, has some major flaws. However, it is not the only way that it can continue to evolve. The first generation of managed care began with placing some limits on benefits. These were deductibles, coinsurance, cost sharing, utilization review, and often, second surgical opinions. This first stage of managed care was usually linked to indemnity insurance. The second generation of managed care began with different types of benefits in the system and out of the system, depending on whether the patient used the physicians and the hospitals that were part of the network. The terms utilized are as follows: networks of providers, PPOs, IPAs (Independent Providers Association), MSOs (Medical Services Organizations), and utilization management. As a member of a preferred provider organization (PPO) and a high user of resources as a specialist, the next year this provider may no longer be a part of that group since high utilization of resources has made the specialist an inefficient provider. This means that the provider can no longer practice within that particular managed-care framework. The third generation of managed-care moves to advanced provider selection, patient-care monitoring, and the utilization of quality measures. There has not been much of the latter yet, at least not in the New York metro area. Kaiser Permanente, in California, had done some work with quality control, but for the most part, managed care begins with price sensitivity. Eventually, it may move on to quality issues. This third generation of managed care usually moves into a heavily capitated system. A popular cartoon depicts a downcast physician and reads as follows: "Poor Doctor Morton, he overprescribed and now has to make up the deficit."

Medicaid managed care, in New York State, has now enrolled 15.2 percent of Medicaid recipients. The for-profit plans offered are the following: Aetna, Managed Care, Oxford, and US Health Care. There are two not-for-profits that are not Article 28 sponsors and two that are Article 28 sponsors. The managed-care market penetration for New York City is proceeding rapidly.

In the United States there are currently 545 HMOs enrolling close to 50 million people. About 18 percent of the nation's population is enrolled in some form of a health maintenance organization. Market penetration of HMOs in Minnesota is now over 30 percent, and in California, over 35 percent. Managed-care penetration in California is close to 70 percent. There is little indemnity insurance in that state. The New York HIP (Health Insurance Plan) is the largest HMO in the state. US Health Care enrolls about 300,000 people. Managed care is moving at a tremendous penetration rate. Aetna's rate in New York City is up 103 percent and up 185 percent for the state. The HMO growth is tremendous because business sees it as a less costly way of providing health insurance to employees. Whether or not it is actually a less costly process is still very much debatable.

What then has been the impact of increased managed-care penetration nationally? First of all, there has been a decreased emphasis on tertiary hospitals and the use of specialist physicians. In medical education, the primary care physician is taught to do as much as possible. Routine gynecology and routine psychosocial screening, for instance, can be done within the scope of knowledge and skill of the primary care physician. Managed care directs referral to a specialist only when absolutely necessary. There is an increased emphasis in primary care and the use of delivery systems alternative to that of inpatient care. Nursing home, home health care, and other technologies are recommended in order to reduce the consumption of inpatient services. Nursing homes are particularly good alternatives since they represent cost shifting to another provider.

Looking at the consequence of this development, in New York City, we can see that those covered by Medicare, as an example, use about four days of service per thousand. In the United States, the national average is lower. New York City's rate of utilization has always been higher than the national average. In California, however, that national figure is cut in half. For those enrolled in HMOs in California, the figure is even lower than that. Is the need for inpatient service utilization going down? Is it because the heaviest users—the medicare-aged enrollees under managed care—are "managed" not to use the hospitalization resources? Does this mean that these people are healthier? The answer to all these questions is that we do not know as yet. In New York City, the average person below the age of 65 who has indemnity insurance uses about 1.2 days per year. In the United States, the national average for that group is less than one day. In California, it is slightly over half a day.

In the California HMOs, the figure is only half a day per year. The effect of managed care on hospital utilization is clear. The need for social workers in hospitals who only perform discharge planning will, therefore, not be doing great in the future under this system since the rate of inpatient care is rapidly shrinking.

In the development of the stages of managed care in any geographical area, if the penetration rate is less than 15 percent, the hospitals will usually dominate the system. The New York metro area is just at this border. Currently, it is at the 15 percent penetration rate, but is about to get higher. The hospitals are dominating the system, but are giving way to the HMOs within the hospital system. Eventually, at stage three, when there is between 30 and 40 percent of market penetration, the HMOs and other parts of the managed-care system take over and dominate health care in that geographic area. When there is over 40 percent market penetration, the HMOs eventually own everything, including the hospitals.

What does this portend for the future of social work in health care? Some predictions are that within a five- to ten-year period about 75 percent of all health care will be controlled by less than 250 health care organizations, if the current trend continues. There may be some truly integrated systems providing prevention services through nursing home care home-supports, hospice care, and other forms of assisted living, but these will be interdependent and will attempt to cooperate with each other. Some of these systems will be led by HMOs, others will be led by hospitals, and some will have combined leadership. Many insurance companies will actually run health care services, and others will pool their lives and form special company-owned businesses.

What will happen to Blue Cross/Blue Shield? New York City may be the site of the first example of a drastic change. The Blues in New York will shrink from about 69 current plans down to about 35 plans. Some of the Blues want to leave the system because of certain restrictions that do not allow them to compete effectively in the marketplace. Many small hospitals will merge with larger ones and larger health care systems. This is already beginning to happen. There are, today, four such systems in New York City. They are the New York University system, which is the largest; the New York Cornell Hospital system; the Mt. Sinai System; and one currently in process of development, the Presbyterian system. The Catholic hospital system will also emerge to become another dominant one in this area. The Mt. Sinai Hospital system, as an example, has made affiliations with hospitals in Nassau and Suffolk counties, all five New York City boroughs, Westchester, Putnam, and Colombia counties, and as far south as Palm Beach, Florida.

Many people who work for large corporations in the United States do not seem to give much thought to the cost of their health care. One popular cartoon depicts a person saying, "I have a headache, I went in for an MRI, and the doctor gave me some aspirin." Such attitudes contribute to the rationale for managed care in this society. People who work for small companies and have an HMO plan have it, somewhat, more inconvenient. Those who are self-employed or unemployed report negative responses when applying for medical insurance. When asked about their illness history and admitting to just having one cold during the last five years, they often hear, in response, "Sorry, we don't insure people with a history of illness." Unfortunately, this happens to be more true than we know. The few lucky individuals who can get an insurance company to write a policy for them may then have to cut back on a few minor things, such as food and rent, since the cost of individual insurance is, ordinarily, high. However, they feel fortunate to be covered.

Managed care is still in many respect in its infancy. There is a set of questions that one needs to ask in order to follow, understand, and analyze the future impact of this development. First, do some managed care models perform better than others? We do not know the answer. Second, are managed care organizations committed to providing services to low-income persons and those with complex and costly medical problems? Some are and some are not. Third, does managed care weaken the position of traditional health care providers, particularly, teaching hospitals, specialty hospitals, and community-based providers? Fourth, does managed care threaten physicians' professional autonomy and compromise their ability to provide high-quality medical care? Fifth, are managed care organizations delivering high-quality medical care? There may not be agreement on exactly what "high quality" is. We do not have the answer to that question either. Sixth, does the manner in which physicians are paid affect the quality of care? For example, if physicians are paid not to use medical resources, does that affect quality? Seventh, does sponsorship for the organization, i.e., for-profit or not-for-profit, affect the commitment to high-quality care for all patients? Eighth, are managed-care plans truly more efficient than fee-for-service plans? The Office of Management and Budget in 1992, in its study of managed care, concluded that they are not more efficient. Managed-care plans show better results because they attempt to limit their enrollment to healthier people. It is that factor which seems to account for the slightly reduced cost difference.

What then is the effect of this reform phenomenon on social work practice? First, there is now a changed model of illness. That model is moving away from a singular biological cause. The head of the National Institute of Health, Dr. Varmus still suggests, however, that most resources should go into the biological base of illness rather than the psychobiosocial base. Even he, however, seems to be moving on that issue. There is a discernible move to an integrated model, in which social work can have a greater contribution than that of a purely biological model. The aim of treatment or cure seems to be moving to amelioration and functional intervention, which is episodic. Most social workers in health care currently work in inpatient settings and see their clients in these settings. In the very near future, however, they will need to move into continuous-care systems. The role of the patient, also, is moving from a passive recipient into one more active. In order for these changes to become institutionalized, social workers must begin to learn more about social epidemiology since the changes will involve dealing with large populations. Managed care enrolls populations not individuals. Social workers' ability to look at populations, as compared to the current denominator function, becomes a crucial factor. Therefore, health status, epidemiology, and social epidemiology must be added to the curriculum of schools of social work. Although it is important to treat health needs, mostly social workers in the future will be supporting the functional needs of people as they progress through the life cycle.

Some examples of "social epidemiological data" relevant to the function of the social worker can be identified in the following: A 60-year-old male has an average life expectancy of 20.6 more years, while a female of that age has 26.5 years. At the age of 100, there is still a mean average life expectancy of 2.3 years for a male and 3.6

years for a female. This means that some people may live longer and others less. Given that some will be living longer, what do we know about this elderly population that can be helpful to them in the management of their later years? They now comprise about 12 percent of the population. However, they use one-third of all physician time and account for 40 percent of all hospital admissions. They also consume 25 percent of all medications sold. One-third of all personal health expenditures are consumed by this group. It is also a population that keeps many social workers in their jobs and creates new social work positions. In addition, 50 percent of the average lifetime health care expenses are incurred in the last two years of life, and 60 percent of that figure is incurred in the last six weeks of life, with seemingly little life quality benefit for most people.

Is the same figure true for the elderly's increase in the use of nonhospital services? There has been a 61 percent increase in the elderly's use of nursing homes and a 36 percent increase in their use of community services. Medicare home health care has increased by 47 percent. What is the risk of needing nursing home care? People who die between the ages of 65 and 74 have a 17 percent probability that they will use a nursing home sometime in the period before death. Those who die between the ages of 75 and 84 have a 36 percent probability of using a nursing home. For those who die between the ages of 85 and 94, there is a 60 percent probability of nursing home use. The two fastest growing age groups in the United States, currently, are men over 75 and women over 85. Can social workers, in any way, effect these probability statistics? There is good reason to believe that they can.

Disability is another major area for expanding social work services. The risk of disability increases with age. Those between age sixty-five and seventy-four stand a 6 percent change of becoming disabled. Those between age seventy-five and eighty-five have a 13 percent chance. Over the age of eighty-five, there is a 40 percent chance of becoming disabled. Think of the implications if one is doing population-focused work for prevention, home support, and teaching health. Think of the implications for social work intervention. The linking of social agencies to the health care system is one major function for the social worker in the near future.

What then are the future most promising social work domains in the health industry? The first is work with the chronically ill who need help not only as inpatients in the hospital, but even more so in the community. This involves a transfer of the focus of work from the hospital to the physician's office and to the concept of "health care without walls," namely, the ambulatory setting. Most important, the change will require service in the neighborhoods where people live. The chronically ill are vulnerable and require social service assistance. The aging population, who utilize so much of the health resource, can be helped to learn how to use less and still improve the quality of their lives. They can learn how to reduce the risks for disability and the subsequent need for expensive and sometimes dehumanizing nursing home care. Social workers should test the adequacy of their capabilities in these areas and should respond to the need for health care to be located within the community. In every community social workers can contribute to enhancing the programs for improving community health.

As an example, the Mt. Sinai Hospital was the recipient, along with one of its health care partners called Settlement Health in East Harlem, of a grant for cardiovascular risk reduction in East Harlem. For three years, an attempt was made to get Latinos and African Americans to reduce their intake of whole milk, meat, pork, and salt. The three-year experiment failed miserably. The school system was involved to no avail. Finally, one resident in a discussion asked why the bodega owners were not involved. That is the place where most residents actually purchased their food. A major education program with bodega owners was then instituted. The bodega owners were convinced that it would be a good idea to participate in this education program and were promised that it would not hurt their marketing. They were also guaranteed that they would earn the same income. In order words, they were insured for a reimbursement, if they lost money because of participating in the program for educating people to eat in a healthier fashion. Once having involved this group, good things started to happen. The school education program, the exercise program, and the smoke-enders program began to show some significant results. The entire program became a profoundly successful one and had a major impact on cardiovascular risk reduction in that geographical area. This was followed by a major federal grant to study how to reduce stroke in that same population. Social workers played a major role in these activities and effectively participated in other programs that truly enhanced the health of people in the community.

Do social workers belong in the offices of primary care physicians in large numbers? Most patients who enter primary care offices are healthy. Therefore, from a public health perspective, they are usually not at high risk. There are screening devices which are sensitive and specific that can determine the people at risk. Such high-risk people can be identified and worked with since they will eventually be heavy users of health care resources. This is why the health care system including managed care will pay social workers to perform such functions. They will pay because it is in everybody's interest to do so. Social workers need to work together with other health officials to develop and perfect such screening instruments. A number of these are already in use and a new one, reported in the *Journal of Social Work and Health Care*, was developed by Berkman and colleagues (1996).[1] This is an excellent new screening instrument based upon some of the previous work of Rehr, Berkman, and Rosenberg. This instrument focuses on primary-care screening with the elderly. It does an excellent job of identifying those older people in need of care.

Social workers will still be performing transition planning in inpatient settings, but there will be fewer workers performing that function. This will take place as patients are followed from the community care facility to the inpatient setting rather than by waiting at the hospital for them to arrive.

Those social workers who enter the management and planning track will discover that there will, probably, not be departments of social work in hospitals in the manner that we now know them. In the future, social workers in health care will be independent, self-directed practitioners. They will probably be carefully supervised, in the first few years, and then they will be expected to become responsible to their respective teams in a matrix format. They will be responsible to the profession perhaps, through a social work director, but there will not be the layers of management that exist today. Social work managers will have to be crossfunctional. They will manage a number of human service endeavors within the health care system.

The health care system of the future cannot function effectively unless it is linked to social service agencies. In this domain, social workers are the most qualified professionals to create and implement this form of linkage. However, most social agencies are small in comparison to the unusually huge size of health systems. The health care system can easily dominate the agencies and if medicalization of social services results, this would be disastrous. Therefore, the future linkage must involve a partnership, one that respects the unique nature of community social service agencies. This is a dilemma that needs to be closely monitored in the years ahead.

Social workers who become directors of health care organizations usually have special experience and expertise. As a group, they seem to be creative and innovative, and they are usually recognized by the management of health care system as such. They are, currently, being utilized for these qualities. There are numerous examples, particularly from California, which demonstrate that in the face of drastic cuts, social work first was reduced in numbers, but later increased beyond anyone's expectations. This happened because social workers proved that by using this community model that they had something special to contribute to the health care system. The Huntington Memorial Hospital, the Kaiser System, the Puget Sound System, and the HMOs in the State of Washington—particularly in Seattle—are excellent examples of this community model and the utilization of social workers.

Several of the health care systems in the New York City area will survive in a very viable partnership with social agencies. Perhaps, it will not be the health care social worker who will perform these functions. The social agency social worker could emerge as the community health care worker. We can no longer function as only part of a single organization with discrete boundaries. If the profession can accept this change and begin to think that way, social work will thrive. This profession has something valuable to offer that is good for the health care system and good for the consumer of the services.

Can social workers compete with other professions for top-level management positions in health care systems? Yes they can.

Mt. Sinai, in New York, is a billion-dollar corporation, and along with a few other people at the top of the management structure, is my position, Senior Vice President.

We are the equivalent of a Fortune 500 Company. Some of my colleagues from other disciplines used to be very ambivalent about treating the poor. But now, they no longer are. They want as many Medicaid patients as they can get to enroll in the Mt. Sinai health system. Am I surprised about this change in attitude? No, it makes financial sense. How can a hospital fill its beds without a base population? Our system needs 250,000 enrolled "lives." The nomenclature now is "lives." Enrollees are no longer called people. In a city like New York, I believe that community benefit standards will be upheld. In other areas, I am not so sure. Where will the uninsured and the undocumented aliens get help? The emerging health systems are not open to serving those populations; perhaps emergency room services will remain as a last-resort medical treatment. Some hospitals are already closing their emergency rooms. Under the best of conditions, however, that is not a sound use of resources to provide primary care. A national social policy must provide increasing access to health care for all people, and it must provide the ability to pay for this. We do not need more money in health care system to do that. We need to eliminate some of the for-profit policies and some of the inefficient administrative structures. Think of the cost of filling out 7,000 different forms for 2,000 different insurance companies, when one form could suffice. This alone could save 10 to 12 percent of the percent of the cost of health care in this nation, representing $100 million. It could be a tremendous savings. The money is there. We do not need more of the gross national product.

How does managed care affect the psychiatrically ill? Unfortunately, our health system continues a duality of treatment. Managed behavioral health care is in even worse shape than managed general health. A sad example is that of a young woman insured in Massachusetts, utilizing a managed care company. She had a very severe, obsessive-compulsive disorder, and needed to be hospitalized. The managed-care company had an arrangement with only one psychiatric hospital, and would not reimburse her for placement in the special unit in that state at another hospital, which specialized in that disorder. The woman received poor care because of the limitations of the insurance company's plan. Their plan does not advocate for its clients. It advocates only for how much profit it can make. It advocates for cost control, rather than the appropriate utilization of treatment. This is far more apparent in managed behavioral health care. Behavioral health managed care is very scary. Our most vulnerable populations are the psychiatrically ill. I predict that they will continue to get poorly treated under managed health care. This is a critical issue, which deserves much discussion and requires special attention.

NOTE

1. Berkman, Barbara, Susan Shearer, W. June Simmons, Monika White, Mark Robinson, Suzanne Sampson, William Holmes, Deborah Allison, and Judith A. Thomson. "Ambulatory elderly patients of private care physicians: Functional, psychosocial, and environmental predictors of need for social work care management." *Social Work and Health*, 22 (3), 1996, pp. 1-20.

Chapter 10

The Substitution Phenomenon of Professionals in the Health Care Industry

Lorna S. McBarnette

The future of all health professionals and the future of social work as a profession within the health care industry are clearly integrally related. Those in health professions that are not fully clinically oriented must prepare themselves to carefully measure and evaluate the outcomes of their interventions as part of a collective process of developing strategies necessary to survive in this new era of health care reform. The term survival may sound "harsh" and prematurely pessimistic; however, it emanates from the most current health management literature. Indeed, it appears that survival is one of the issues social workers discuss in their national meetings and conferences.

For many years, health professionals have been strongly supported by government, business, and the public. Because of the important roles they have played in matters concerning life, health, and death, they were trusted to serve and to incorporate the latest in knowledge and technology into their professional work. Participants in the latest round of health care reform discussions, which have focused on the rising costs of care, as a priority—higher than access and quality issues—have identified health professionals with the problems of rising costs and poor quality. The market for health care has become increasingly turbulent and unpredictable, causing serious rivalry within and among professional groups. Large health delivery service delivery organizations, potential substitute professions, and insurers have begun to challenge the prevailing practices and attitudes in the division of health care labor.[1] Professional groups are invading each other's traditional work roles and scope of practice, and challenging long-held tenets of professional practice.

Health professionals currently find themselves in adversarial rather than allied roles vis-á-vis health insurance companies and hospitals—both struggling to capture and retain market shares in the face of ever-increasing competition. After enjoying decades of relative insulation from external economic and political scrutiny, many health professionals find themselves working for the new players in the health arena—vertically and horizontally integrated business enterprises judged by their ability and capacity to compete in an economic marketplace. Workers observe that they are being treated as "inputs" into the product called health care. These large health care corporations and conglomerates show a preference for routinization and rationalization of professional work in order to demystify, manage, and control the work of health professionals. In this context, many professional groups have expressed concern that they are being "deprofessionalized."

The health care environment has become more complex than ever, and this complexity has caused professionals and their associations to reconsider their relationships with third-party payers, hospitals, government agencies, the public, other professions, and even members of their own group. Some observers have cited a need for professional associations to develop strategies to position their profession in relation to external demands.[2] A major function of professional associations, according to Price and Del Polito, is to assess current and emerging trends affecting the environment that impact on their members activities.[3]

The challenges are greater for some professions than others. For example, the protracted struggle among social workers, psychiatrists, and psychologists over domain definition and the appropriate division of labor in mental health remains unresolved.

The professional association, in the case of social workers, must examine the professional preparation of social workers for their defined roles, the current public policies that enhance or impede their professional growth and development, and opportunities for effective advocacy that move the profession forward.

Every profession evolves from an academic foundation; therefore, an important role of the professional association is to reinforce the substance of the academic curriculum which fosters research concerning the theoretical foundations of practice, the efficacy of treatment modalities, new techniques, and other variables.[4] Whereas, the abstract nature of professional knowledge strengthens a profession's ability to avoid external quality assessments. For example, the indetermination of a profession's knowledge base can become too extreme, prompting external intervention, on the basis that the knowledge has no verifiable utility. *Social work, in the eyes of some observers, suffers from this problem.* The efforts of major purchasers of health care to find cheaper substitutes will no doubt increase, and just as many other professionals are battling against the use of substitutes, social workers must implement strategies to avoid competition with practitioners from other professions, with consumer self-help, and with other forms of substitutes in order to avoid dilution of their profession. The need is to create the following:

- Clear and relevant standards of practice
- Consistent credentialing procedures
- Relevant continuing education programs
- Faculty development programs

The overlapping boundaries with psychiatry and psychology will continue to cause problems for social workers unless they arrive at a clearer professional definition and a set of standards that individual practitioners are expected to meet. In the case of social workers in medical organizations, the need for clarification is urgent. There must be a well-planned effort to delineate the scope of practice and create professional boundaries. This step is central to determining competence and to developing and measuring outcomes. The question of measurement is key in any discussion of the challenges facing social workers. The inability to measure the outcomes of social work intervention and the abstract nature of professional knowledge make the profession ripe for substitution.

THE CHANGING HEALTH CARE ENVIRONMENT

Demographic changes, economic conditions, cultural force, and governmental policies, combined with the knowledge sectors of our society are affecting the work of health professionals and creating uncertainty about their roles and contributions in the short and long term.

Health care expenditures in the U.S. approximate 14.0 percent of the Gross National Product (GNP), rising annually between 1950 and 1990, at a fairly steady rate. Business entities—employers, have become concerned about the proportion of income they spend on health benefits, and consumers experienced health care expenditures rising from 4.2 percent of adjusted personal income in 1965 to 5.1 percent in 1989.[5] Additionally, between 31 and 36 million Americans had no health insurance on any given day in 1980, and many more were underinsured.[6]

The characteristics of the health care environment changed rapidly because of the cost, quality, and access issues that are being discussed with an eye toward reform. These changes included the initiation of nonlocal, multilayered authority structures, the replacement of traditional physician/administrator/board structures, and the convergence of organizational structural forms, goals, and performance irrespective of for-profit or not-for-profit status. New organizational forms have also arisen: PPOs, HMOs, ambulatory surgical centers, complicated networks and affiliation arrangements, and an array of new products.

Despite the unprecedented change, organizational innovation, and experimentation, there have been organizational failures, occurring in a financial environment that is out of control. Mick and others attribute these failures to events such as prospective reimbursement linked with a case-mix methodology known as Diagnosis-Related Groups (DRG); the availability and infusion of technology; rate-setting commissions that constrain organizational discretion, and the redundant capacity in hospitals as a result of decreasing inpatient utilization.[7] Market failures actually force organizations to rethink their strategies and look for ways of improving their ability to create and sustain competitive advantages.

THE ORGANIZATION
OF THE MEDICAL CARE SECTOR

The medical care sector is organized differently from other sectors involving complex work. Parsons and others stressed the importance of professional occupations within the sector. They emphasized the central role played by professionals in defining the nature and division of the work to be done, in setting standards for evaluating performance, and in determining appropriate control and support structures.[8] Much has been written about professional occupations with changing foci over the years. Throughout, the sustaining focus has been on identifying characteristics that distinguish professions from other occupations. Current thinking suggests that professional practice is based on the following:

1. A body of general, systematic knowledge.
2. Professionals asserting the need for autonomy in decision making, i.e., protection from nonprofessional controls.
3. Professional norms that espouse altruism or a service orientation.

These assumptions about professional characteristics posited that a single generic model covered all professional occupations. Disagreements arose only around the number, definition, and relative importance of the distinguishing factors. Abbott points out that these early observers were prone to emphasize the assumptions of a generic model because they were looking at one profession—medicine—and one context—the United States. Another problem with these earlier analyses, and the proposed generic is the underlying notion of ahistoricity—a tendency to deemphasize changes over time.[9]

In recent times, analysts have begun to take a more careful look at differences within and among professional occupations and to examine changes over time in their distinctive features. Examinations of relations among varying professional occupations, changes over time in the process of professionalization, and differences related to place, method, and time of their development have revealed a plethora of differing concerns among groups. Earlier researchers emphasized the functionalist role in professional practice, assuming that professional stature arose as solutions to problems. General, systematic knowledge was required to deal with unusually complex problems, collegial controls were necessary because nonprofessionals could not evaluate the quality of the work being performed, and altruistic norms were needed to ensure that professionals would not exploit dependent clients.[10]

As a society, we have come to recognize the benefits associated with professional forms to the professionals themselves, and recent works focus on the process by which professional occupational groups acquire power to enforce their monopoly positions and escape external controls. Abbott and others highlight the devising of ideological arguments that emphasize the importance of the services provided and the complexity and uncertainty of the work performed.[11] The acquisition of state support for exclusive jurisdiction over specified types of work or occupational titles is today a fundamental factor in gaining professional power, title protection, and prestige. So, we see many other professional groups taking the route to licensure as a means of protecting their titles and scope of practice. Occupational licensing is the most visible method of establishing an occupational monopoly. It is the process by which government grants exclusive official permission, sustained by law, to eligible individuals to work in a particular occupation. The problem is that whereas, licensure always offers title protection—exclusive use of a title—it does not always protect the scope of practice. For example, social workers in some states are in the position where only a licensed person may use the title *certified social worker*, but a nonlicensed person is not prevented offering the same services to the public. This leaves the profession without protection in terms of the industry's efforts at substitution.

There is even a larger system of privately controlled credentialing in the United States. This occurs under the auspices of the professions themselves, through their associations. A certificate is awarded to a qualified candidate, usually after having completed a specified course of study and practice at an accredited professional school and sometimes after having passed an examination. Even though a state may not have laws establishing licenses for certified social workers, social workers can qualify for certification through their own profession. Unfortunately, all forms of occupational credentialing—public or private—have a critical weakness, according to Eliot Friedson: ". . . they may be able to restrict or narrow the supply of qualified professionals, but they cannot, in and of themselves, control demand."[12] To illustrate, there is relatively little value to be a licensed social worker in a state where consumers seeking services are free to visit practitioners who cannot legally use the title but can offer what appear to be the same services. Occupational credentialing without appropriate standards, scope of practice, and title protection constitutes a limited advantage in a marketplace in which buyers and sellers are free to exercise choice.

STATE-PROFESSIONAL RELATIONSHIPS

Government plays a multifaceted role in its relationships with health care and other professionals. The backing of the state is necessary to secure a monopoly market position for an occupational group. This type of support involves giving exclusive access to an area of practice, jurisdiction over a set of activities, or, sometimes only the right to use an occupational title. However, the state can act in other ways. By subsidizing research and training activities, or by stimulating the creation of particular types of provider arrangement, e.g., Health Maintenance Organizations or managed-care arrangements, it proscribes the terms and conditions under which some professionals work. The state can also restrict employment in specified positions to those with particular professional certification, and even more significant, it can insist that only those with appropriate certification be paid with state tax dollars for services provided.[13] Of significance, in terms of state role, the more powerful professions—such as medicine—have been allowed to share in the exercise of legitimate state power in a variety of ways: setting standards, drafting legislation, or serving on implementation or review groups established or mandated to administer or oversee publicly funded and mandated programs. Looking at these arrangements from the perspective of power theorists, one can surmise that they are subject to abuse although important benefits can be derived from self-regulation. Some professional groups' attempts at self-regulation and gatekeeping have not been successful. Weak professions, according to Friedson, "can only use moral suasion and the issuance of official standards that have none of the force of organized institutional credentialing." An example of this is the series of professional standards for social work in various settings issued as policy statements by the National Association of Social Workers. Among stronger professions, such as medicine and dentistry, recommendations become the basis for establishment of legal requirements.

STRATEGIES TO MINIMIZE THE CHALLENGES

The challenges to social work in this new health care environment are great ones. One of the critical issues is the difficulty in measuring the outcomes of social work practice. This inability to measure successful outcomes, however, is really no different than the current arguments about primary care versus specialty care in medicine. The federal government has indicated to physicians that it will now pay more to those who utilize their skills in the delivery of primary health care as opposed to those who utilize their technical skills in specialties. Although a different context, this concept could be related to the position of social workers in health care.

The national leadership in the profession of social work needs to create a context for the societal revaluing of this profession. If the nation can indeed revalue the role of primary-care physicians, then this concept should apply to other professions that exercise conceptual skills in the delivery of services as opposed to those that use technical skills. The abstract nature of professional knowledge often strengthens a profession's ability to avoid quality-assessment games and external controls. The determination of a profession's knowledge base can be of immeasurable help. If the public has difficulty comprehending what social workers do or the curriculum by which they are educated, it is understandable that they will not value it. Is the social work professional curriculum too indeterminate? Does it need to become more rigorous? Does it also need to be standardized on a national level so that everyone can recognize the end product? Certainly, those who administer and make policy for the health care industry need such understanding and clarification. When soft definitions and indeterminate knowledge becomes too extreme, as may be the case in social work, it invites external intervention on the basis that there is no verifiable utility of the service performed. The professional knowledge base as reflected in the practice in social work can raise serious questions about such verifiable utility of the profession.

The major purchasers of health care will continue to search for cheaper substitutes for service providers. This trend will no doubt expand to other health professionals who are battling against the use of substitutes. Social workers must quickly devise and implement strategies to prevent such substitutions, since they are already taking place by managed-care companies and by some hospitals.

A major difficulty is the constant interchangeable use of the terms "health care" and "medical care." In the medical care paradigm, people get sick, they enter the system, there is an intervention, and they either get well or die. That is the classic medical model. The health care model proposes that the professionals try to keep people well and intervene in the social processes that potentially might make them ill. As we intervene in the social processes, it is possible to influence the responses to the illness experience. We attempt also to create a social climate that helps people to remain well once they have overcome the clinical experience. This second model of "health care" helps in understanding and valuing the contribution of social workers since that is exactly what social workers in health care can do. Competition with the medical profession and the issue of medical clinical intervention as opposed to social intervention, however, continues to plague the health professions. The changes we are seeing in nomenclature, such as calling one setting a "medical center" as opposed to an "academic health center," are significant, particularly in a university environment. The implications of such organizational changes, which appear on the surface to be benign, send out very strong political messages that encourage organizational policies and practices calculated to diminish the role of social work in health care.

THE ENVIRONMENT

The environment of health care, as has been indicated, is changing rapidly. The role of government, cultural values, economic conditions, and political factors are clearly affecting the status of health care professionals. These are also creating uncertainty for professionals about their roles and their contributions. This is all being done under the guise of cost containment, with particular concern about the cost of health care insurance to corporate business. Concern is also being expressed about the cost to the public sector of the uninsured and the underinsured. The policy decisions are being made by people far removed from bedsides, the clinic, the patient's home, or the academic health center. Health professionals have remained significantly silent when budget cuts, substitutions, and other policy changes have been made in areas that produce great vulnerability to them. They need to take a more activist stance when such things occur. Clients who use the health care services of social workers also should be mobilized to make articulate demands for such services and must be organized in order to take such action.

Some of the changes taking place, or being projected, are, of course, positive ones and should be encouraged. At the federal and state policy levels, however, there is not enough response from health professionals who should be encouraging discussion about public health and the importance of social interventions in the quality-of-life issues. The public health reform movement emphasizes a strong focus on social health issues along with clinical and medical health concerns. It should be understood that if national health care policy does not focus on social issues as well, it is not only social workers who will be affected, but many other professionals as well. The medical model that will emerge will be much more costly to manage. The dollars to support such a model of medical care will result in fewer other services being affordable items within the system.

New organizational structures are beginning to develop. Multiple layers of policy and administration are replacing the traditional relationships between administrators, boards, and physicians. Major conversions of structural forms, goals, and performance criteria are now taking place in both for-profit and not-for-profit health care organizations. New organizational forms, such as PPOs, HMOs, and ambulatory surgical centers are emerging. Many represent complex networks and agreements, providing an array of new products that all seem to cry out for strong case management to help a client in working through these complex mazes. Knowledge about and skill in dealing with social processes, public health services, and feelings of people within organizational structures are all areas in which social workers have historically gained the greatest amount of community experience. However, the trend now is to eliminate reimbursement for these types of social services. In effect, the social services in health care seem destined for potential elimination. This trend has been observable now for several years, yet the advocacy stance of health care professionals to counter this development has been at best a weak one.

Many organizational failures in health care have occurred due to the financial environment seeming to be out of control. These failures have been linked to policies like DRGs. Supply often creates demand in the health care field just as it does in other market areas. Every time a new technology is created, there is pressure to make somebody use it. A great deal of funding is going into the high-tech arena, some of it unnecessarily. A great deal of intervention in professional medical functioning is also now taking place, i.e., utilization reviews, quality assessments, appropriateness review, etc. Physicians are hard pressed—as are other professionals—to monitor these developments and to raise the questions about the appropriateness of the professional behavior involved in their utilization. The medical care sector is not organized in the same way as other sectors that are involved in highly complex activity. Studies of professions within the health care sector seem to emphasize the limited role played by the professional in defining the nature of his or her work and the role in defining a proper division of labor. This may be the most critical factor when one examines the rising cost of health care. The medical care system has been designed to revolve around the physician. He or she determines the kind of clinical work that needs to be done. The professional bias today seems to be toward high-tech intervention. Malpractice insurance as a cost factor has also contributed heavily to this emphasis on expensive diagnostic procedures. Another factor related to poor outcomes is that other professional health care staff who have been trained to deal with sequelae of these interventions are not appropriately brought into the scene in timely fashion.

In this era of a highly complex, multiorganizational health care system, the case management function becomes a critical one. Who then is the most appropriately trained professional to perform case management? The answer depends, of course, on how case management is defined. Comprehensive case management entails a concern for the clients' survival and effective and efficient utilization of services resulting in positive outcomes. This must involve the use of intervention in the social processes, as well as ensuring that the sutures were put in competently after the surgical procedure. Social services such as housing, counseling, job placement, family adjustment, and income maintenance are critical to successful outcomes, yet these seem not to be appropriately valued in the medical care sector.

PROFESSIONALISM

Professional practice is based upon a body of general systematic knowledge. Professionals assert the need for autonomy in decision making and in protection from nonprofessional controls. The professional norms usually espouse altruism or a service orientation. Talcott Parsons described the profession of medicine in these terms many years ago. This, however, describes all professions. Disagreements only arise concerning the number of characteristics identified by Parsons and how they are defined. It has been pointed out that the general assumption is ahistoric in that it fails to look at how professions have developed over time. The immediate time and place that the definition relates to does not help to predict what may happen in the future.

It is important to discuss not only generalities among the professions, but commonalties as well. Education for the professions should consider the development of a basic core of knowledge and values to which every professional should be exposed. There are additional ongoing discussions about specialists versus generalists. At the same time, given the division of labor concept, the significant differences between professions must also be considered. If we do such rethinking, the result may be richer jobs and fewer job titles rather than fewer workers.

There is much to be done in terms of reengineering jobs and educating professionals so educated people may have a fuller plate and not be dissatisfied with what they do because of boundary limitations. There is a need to challenge the existing curricula of professional programs in the health area. Are these programs too ambitious or are they too limited? Are graduates prepared to deal with reality issues in the profession at the entry level and beyond? If not, what changes in the curriculum are needed? Education in all professions struggles with these questions. Some are denying the challenge; others are accepting it. Physical therapy and occupational therapy are occupations experiencing a national dialogue about similarity versus differences. Both sides are discovering that there seem to exist more similarities than differences. However, the professional organizations struggle against the notion of cross training. What should emerge in that example is a bigger and better rehabilitation specialist who can earn a lot more money and be a lot more productive than the model being proposed by the two competing groups. The issue seems to be a similar one for psychologists and social workers. Rather than scrambling up the ladder and kicking the other down, and rather than attempting to shut the other out of licensing, there is a need to broaden the boundaries as opposed to narrowing them.

CREDENTIALING ISSUES

There are, approximately, 35 health professions now licensed in one or more states. These include, among others, chiropractors, environmental health engineers, optometrists, pharmacists, physical therapists, etc. Social workers are licensed in some states and certified in others. Is there a difference between licensure and certification? There is, and social workers need to become aware of what that difference means. In New York, the state agencies have been an interesting partner in this issue of professional competition. The state gives and the state can take away. Although social workers are certified in many states, the certification has come about because they are performing certain functions that the state will pay for only if performed by a certified or licensed professional. However, such policies can change easily. If an important state official disagrees with a policy, a meeting is called, which can result in a recommendation for a change to the legislature. Certification represents recognition of academic credentials, a gateway to the entry level; it indicates that one is minimally qualified to perform certain functions. Licensure establishes a title and a field of practice, one that no one else may use for practice or title without the license. A scope of practice is defined, including the things that the licensed professional may do that no one else can do. Significant reciprocity is usually granted as the professional moves from place to place in pursuit of the profession. The groups that have licensure struggle to protect it from other groups who may want it. Licensure is critical to a profession, and there is a cost to achieving it. However, it seems to be worth the struggle to the professionals. Leaders in social work should ask themselves, Why have other professions been so quick to move toward licensure and so eager to protect it, and why have some groups been precluded from licensure? How can a scope of practice for social work be created and defined that can address this critical issue. The social work profession and its national organizations must make this question a priority. Are there differences between the basis upon which psychologists in the state are licensed and social workers only certified? This question needs to be asked, given the similarities in functions between the two professions.

There is also the phenomenon of state government, which can restrict employment in specified positions for those with particular professional certification. Even more significant is that the state can insist that only those with appropriate certification be paid with tax dollars for the services provided. In health care this is becoming an increasingly significant issue. Managed care, cost reduction, HMOs, and other factors clearly indicate that payment procedures and eligibility requirements will change if the move toward substitutions continues. There will probably be a scaling down of the credentials of people who produce certain services rather than a "scaling up." Dismissing the profession of social work from the health care system can simply be done by declaring that there will be no reimbursement for counseling or case management services. It would be easy to posit the proposition that there is no clinical intervention in the counseling function and that there is no negative potential if counseling services were eliminated. There is indeed still a serious lack of understanding in the health care area of needs that are not physical and do not produce physical pain or bleeding. In this quest for substitutions for professions in health care, a great deal of damage may occur in the quest for cost reduction.

The substitution issue is occurring in many of the health professions. It may be instructive to consider the field of nursing, which since the days of Florence Nightingale has been seen as an ironclad profession. Nursing has made the same mistakes that social work is about to make. There have been too many gateways into the profession. Four or five educational models existed in nursing—all which could lead to a license. This leads to questioning the nature and content of the various curricula. The nursing profession strategically created a very loose scope of practice. The descriptive language suggests that the nurse can do almost everything from scrubbing floors to brain surgery. Nurses may not have intended it that way, but others who are attempting to rationalize the field of nursing within a context of health care are confused.

Today in academic medical centers, there is serious discussion of job redesign and job engineering. Pieces of what was supposed to be in the scope of nursing practice are now disappearing. It is claimed by the "reengineers" that these functions should never have been in the scope of nursing practice at all. Certain functions are claimed to be too simplistic for the level of current training, particularly, on the graduate degree level. Does one need a master's degree to make a bed? Care needs to be taken that as curriculum changes are made, job descriptions match the change also. Otherwise, the charges leveled are that professional training programs are overeducating for current positions. It was posed that the nursing shortage could be solved by putting more money into the system, by doing more counseling, or by improving the integrity of the examination. A great deal of money was spent to increase the enrollment in nursing schools in New York State, for example. At that time, the state was recording that large numbers of nursing jobs remained unfilled. A study by the Academy of Medicine raised the question of why so many nurses left the field. The study concluded that nurses did not leave; rather, they were not being hired. Other people were being hired instead. The total number of required jobs was filled. Some 500 nursing jobs vacancies existed. Was there a natural shortage, or were nurses becoming too expensive? At that time, we were witnessing a move by the nursing profession to impose higher standards. They were making the same demands as physicians traditionally have demanded for their profession. Nurses were demanding that they be treated as professionals. Many physicians had a difficult time accepting this, and the controversy was seen as disturbing the workplace environment. Therefore, organizational policymakers began to hire people who were easier to deal with. This phenomenon is part of the political conditions that currently exist. For the first time in seven years, we have unemployed nurses. The demand today is for some other kind of worker at a lower level that would fit into the authority system of the organization. The handwriting on the wall of the health care industry makes it clear that other health professions will be similarly affected.

The legal system seems to condone the practice of substitution. Because the issue of malpractice remains an important one, there is a move to a system of institutional licensure. This suggests that organizations should decide how to credential people in their own organizations. This means that the organization can delineate their professional privileges from inside of the organization. Therefore, the institution can define by decree what specific behavior is acceptable, thus making malpractice liability no longer an issue. One wonders how the health professions and their national standards can survive under such circumstances? Institutional licensure is also an issue that is beginning to be debated. There is concern that such a move would cause problems in service quality when organizations move into a cost-reduction mode. No one seems to know exactly how to resolve this issue, and such discussions are proceeding in all the major academic medical centers. If institutional licensure develops, the organization can decide that anyone with a pleasant personality, seemingly capable of talking with people, could be a social worker, and be hired as one. If there are no bad outcomes that can be measured, as a result of such a substitution, there is little that the profession can do about it.

SCIENTIFIC KNOWLEDGE BASE

The scientific basis of practice has now become a critical issue. It seems necessary to create an aura of science even in those practice areas that today are still nebulous and lack hard data to support their knowledge base, despite having an important value base underlying the practice. It is important now to create this scientific knowledge base and to create significant skill in defending professional practice in those professions that are fighting against substitutions. It is possible to achieve this. However, public information material about social work usually gives a general description of the field, listing the various places where social workers practice and the various functions that they perform. These descriptions sometimes include something about the curriculum of professional education. However, the materials never indicate what body of knowledge needs to be mastered and what level of competence needs to be displayed in order to become a professional social worker. What seems to be needed is a model of competency-based education. Competency does not necessarily derive from numerous or large numbers of core courses. There needs to be a way of measuring competency through challenges or in practicum experience which can let people know that graduates are capable of performing specific functions. Of course, this is easier to achieve in professional schools that teach the use of technology. In social work, there are many clinical functions that can be measured. Other professions have greater difficulty. Primary care physicians will face some of these issues. Can we always measure what we do in health care? The federal government recently said to primary care physicians, "Not to worry." They announced that what primary care physicians do is important and even though we can not quite measure the importance in our lifetime, everything will work out in the long term. Therefore, the government is planning to put a lot of money into primary care physician activity. This frame of reference is needed for all the health professions, which we believe will have good outcomes even though the practice cannot be measured today, as long as there is a commitment to work toward measurement. The investment in moving toward measurement and validating the body of knowledge must be undertaken as quickly as possible. If we believe that this has a chance of working for social workers, then it is important to lobby for this opportunity. Lobbying is sometimes called "educating the legislature." As professionals, we need to spend more time doing this because legislators in the last analysis make the policy decisions that affect how health professionals can practice.

One graphic example of substitution is what took place in the early 1960s. The New York City Welfare Department decided that it was not functioning well. The public was unhappy, the Mayor was unhappy, and the easiest group to blame it on was the social workers. At that time, the deprofessionalization of social workers took place in the public welfare department. The government simply changed entry-level qualifications, downgrading what was expected of the performance of social workers, and hired an entirely new breed of workers into the system, workers who bore no resemblance to professionals. It was done by fiat. *The Daily News* printed three lines about it. The department said, "We did it and nobody turned a hair." Undergraduate-degreed social workers now staff the public welfare system. Looking under the bed for the "man of the house," became synonymous with the social work function. Today, even when the real curriculum is discussed, or the level of commitment needed for professional social work is elucidated, people still describe social workers as "bleeding hearts." It is necessary now to delineate the knowledge and skill base of the profession and to deal with the public question of what is required for professional helping professions.

HEALTH CARE

Health care reform will exacerbate many of these questions. It could also provide an initiative for their resolution. Certainly, managed care policies will require that all professionals in health care will have to become activists if they are to survive in the new health care environment. Faculty in schools of social work have a responsibility, along with social work practitioners in health care, to give national leadership on these issues and alert students to the potential dangers and opportunities. Social workers have a long history of addressing crisis and converting them into opportunities. Time is crucial, and social work will not have a great deal of it to debate these issues in an organized manner.

Social work services in health care cannot continue to function in the traditional manner. Social service delivery in the future will take place in a different fashion. Social workers must stay committed to work with and care for poor and otherwise oppressed people. In order to maximize the effectiveness of their services, social workers must remain strong and viable. The changes in health care structure, financing, and service delivery are proceeding at an extremely rapid rate. The licensed professions, such as medicine and nursing, are positioned to assume new roles and new responsibilities while struggling to survive. Social work must develop an organized strategy to do the same thing. As organizational changes take place within a hospital or in a medical center, the social work profession will be competing heavily with the licensed professions in health care and will need the support of educational programs as well as national organizations in order to maintain its positions. Social workers, therefore, need to know clearly what the other professions in health care are contributing and how they perform their services.

Another issue is how to convince consumers that they need to utilize social work services when the hospital or medical center does not recommend these services. If consumers do not understand the value of the social work services and do not request them, the efficiency factor will be meaningless. Most consumers of health care services at this point in time know little about the contribution that social work can make to their lives, and they do not see social work services as truly important in dealing with physical medical issues. The public image of the social work profession and its information systems need to be upgraded.

Administrators in the health care system who are responsible for running the institutions often do not have the necessary information about the social work contribution and will, therefore, listen to the physicians and the nurses regarding priorities.

There is a small but important amount of research that has documented the effectiveness of social work intervention, particularly in the health care area, but the profession has not effectively utilized this body of knowledge. Given the current conservative political environment, it is understandable that social work has difficulty receiving equal attention. In this respect, the profession may have been its own worse enemy. Social work has significant access to some policy arenas, and members of the profession sit at some of these policymaking tables. Three years ago, for instance, the Congressional Black Caucus had five social workers represented on it. There is a United States Senator with an MSW degree. Why aren't these individuals being lobbied by the profession? Does the profession take for granted that it will be protected?

It should be noted that one important reason for the delay in achieving social work licensing in New York State is the conflict between two groups within the profession regarding the definition of the social work practice to be licensed. One group, represented in the urban areas, strongly supports a narrow clinical definition while the rest of the state supports a significantly broader definition. This is an important issue for social workers in health care particularly as the focus for service may be quickly shifting from the hospital to the larger community. Unlike other health professions, social workers perform many functions that are not clinical. Other functions require a much broader approach to direct social work practice and, therefore, must be covered in a more inclusive definition of direct service. This becomes critical to professional survival since without licensing, reimbursement will not be possible in the future, and without the possibility of third-party reimbursement, many social work functions will be delegated to "substitutes."

Regarding the imperative to validate the effectiveness of social work practice, it is also important to recognize that other professions in health care also function with limited validation of their practice. Even when some people receive "good" medical care, they may not recover from disease or they may die. Yet, rarely are physicians criticized by the public. Medicine, however, does make claims to a science-based body of knowledge, and science is popularly revered. Social work has not yet achieved a science orientation. The art component is still a strong force in the profession's knowledge base. This has value, but does not address the popular commitment to rationality and empiricism. Research in social work is urgently needed, but should not be seen as a total solution to the issues presented. It is important to note, however, that social work, like nursing and teaching, is still seen as a "semi" or "demi" profession. These professions have a common characteristic, namely, their numbers are significantly dominated by women. In this society, this results in lower status and less serious recognition, resulting inevitably in lower reimbursement for services. Because we do not exist in an ordered and rational world, strategies must be developed to recognize and effectively deal with the inconsistencies and prejudices of our society.

Is there resistance among social work practitioners to participate in research activities related to their own practice? Should direct practitioners be expected to devote serious time and energy to research efforts? Should the social work profession create a specialized corps of researchers? Some observers note that the average social work practitioner is too closely focused to the rewards emanating from engagement in human relationship activities. Perhaps the helping relationship is too esoteric to be subjected to rational and empirical scrutiny. In a low-paying profession, how much nonreimbursable time can be devoted to research? Finally, is there resistance to research because practitioners in this profession, like many others, are not ready to face the possible negative findings resulting from careful evaluation of the effectiveness of their practice.

Finally, one must question the impact of the not-for-profit privatization movement currently dominating health care in this nation, which is driven by the major force of the insurance industry. When the fundamental mission of the health care institution is shifted from effective service delivery to maximizing dividends to stock holders, the entire value system and the goals for the institution become displaced. The professions that serve it are also critically affected. Competition is engendered and power struggles develop in order to capture a greater share of the reimbursement dollar, or to maintain the market share. Without a united and cooperative stance, the health professions stand little chance of successfully influencing health care policy.

NOTES

1. Begun, J. W., and R. Lippincott (1993). *Strategic adaptation in the health professions*. San Francisco, CA: Jossey-Bass.

2. Shortell, S. M., E. M. Morrison, and B. Friedman. (1990). *Strategic choices for America's hospitals: Managing change in turbulent times*. San Francisco, CA: Jossey-Bass.

3. Price, G. D., and C. M. Del Polito. (1988). "Role of professional associations in the educational process." In N. Farber, E. J. McTernan, and R. O. Hawkins (eds.). *Allied health education: Concepts, organization, and administration*. Springfield, IL: Charles C Thomas.

4. Ibid, p. 297.

5. Legit, K. R., H. C. Lazenby, S. W. Letsch, and C. Cowan. (1991). National health care spending. *Health Affairs* 10(1), 117-130.

6. Friedman, E. (1991). The uninsured: From dilemma to crisis," *Journal of the American Medical Association*.

7. Mick, S. (1990). *Innovations in health care delivery: Insights for organization theory*. San Francisco: Jossey-Bass.

8. Parsons, T. (1939). The professions and social structure. *Social Forces*, 17, 456-467.

9. Abbott, A. (1988). *The system of professions: An essay on the division of expert labor*. Chicago: University of Chicago Press.

10. Parsons (1939).

11. Abbott (1988).

12. Friedson, E. (1986). *Professional Powers*. Chicago: University of Chicago Press.

13. Scott, R. W., and E. Backman (1989). "Institutional theory and the medical care sector." In Mick (1990).

14. Friedman (1991), p. 85.

Chapter 11

Troubled Preschoolers Making Trouble Later: Is There a Solution?

Judith S. Bloch

Mickey (Bloch, 1971) had a bad start in life. Born out of wedlock, he was placed in a temporary foster home for the first 18 months of his life. At the end of that time, his behavior was already conspicuously deviant and inappropriate. An early psychiatric evaluation was grim. It described three-year-old Mickey as "possibly psychotic" and stated that the prognosis was "guarded." In an attempt to alter his angry, assaultive behavior, exacerbated by early deprivation and isolation, the county social service department placed him with a new foster family, an older, childless couple in their forties. They quickly became devoted and attached to Mickey, their first child; they sought out and placed him in a preschool special education program.

If any criticism were to be made of this couple's care of this hyperactive, unresponsive child, it was that they were too indulgent and permissive. There is no question that the love and care they lavished on him aided and abetted his development and ultimately, along with the school's program, helped Mickey achieve unanticipated but exciting gains.

Carol entered the program as a three-year-old, anxious, angry, disorganized child with a very high activity level. Her limited attention span and learning disabilities required intensive teacher intervention. Her fragile mother, a victim of spousal abuse, had limited parenting skills and limited ability to meet the needs of her three

183

young children. As a result of extensive outreach efforts by the school social worker, the mother began to trust and rely on the parent support, training, and respite that was offered. Mrs. M became more confident and empowered in her ability to manage her children, learned to set reasonable limits, and became more empathic. She came to understand her child's educational needs and became more active in planning for them. When Carol left this program, she spent one year in the district special education program and currently she is being educated in a mainstream classroom.

INTRODUCTION

Presently, this nation has thousands of very young troubled children with similar patterns of antisocial behavior and cognitive, social, educational, and emotional problems. They are already demonstrating behavior that indicates they are at risk of later adult antisocial disorders. There is good reason for communities to be worried about violence and danger in public places as well as personal safety (Eron, 1994; Wallach, 1994) as the numbers of these very young, at-risk children increase.

WHO ARE THE CHILDREN?

A growing population of troubled preschoolers who are likely to become violent juveniles has been identified and described in the literature (Children's Defense Fund, 1994; Public Agenda, 1995). These children have multiple risk factors; they are often neglected and abused, and sometimes neurologically impaired. Some are graduates of a series of unsuccessful foster care placements. The report of The Carnegie Corporation, *Starting Point: Meeting the Needs of Our Youngest Children* (1994), documents a frightening pattern of neglect. It states:

> Compared with most other industrialized countries, the United States has a higher infant mortality rate, a higher proportion of low-birthweight babies, a smaller proportion of babies immu-

nized against childhood diseases, and a much higher rate of babies born to adolescent mothers. Of the 12 million children younger than age three in the United States today, a staggering number are affected by one or more risk factors that undermine healthy development. One in four lives in poverty. One in three victims of physical abuse is a baby younger than age one.

The report concludes that this early adverse environment can compromise a young child's brain function and overall development, placing him or her at greater risk of developing a variety of behavioral and physical difficulties. In some cases, these effects may be irreversible.

Children who do not have at least one adult in their lives who is "crazy about them," and who in turn are not passionately attached and eager to please this adult are not likely to become socialized in acceptable ways (*Young Children*, 1993). It is generally recognized that children of age six must be able to obey adults and follow directions. They are not indifferent to rules and expectations and are responsive to adult approval or disapproval. They have at least one friend, and they find these interpersonal connections reasonably satisfying. That means that they are able to quarrel and reconcile with the significant people in their lives. This kind of social competence is important because children with poor social skills often prompt others to react to them in rejecting and hostile ways. With enough frequency, this pattern will promote the development of a child who is angry, isolated, and without empathic capacity, risk factors for later delinquent behavior. In other words, children ages five or six who demonstrate early and serious problems in attachment and who are already aggressive or destructive are likely to make trouble for others later (Umansky, 1983). Additional characteristics may include the following:

- Behavior problems
- Low IQ scores
- Limited verbal skills
- Learning disabilities
- Reading problems

BLAMING THE MOTHERS

For many of these children, their family picture is bleak. A disproportionate number of parents are poor and single; most did not have prenatal care. The children and families are often without health care, quality child care, or family support systems. Parents are likely to be uninvolved or unable to provide adequate supervision. Poor parental disciplinary patterns and harsh and punitive childrearing practices have been reported. A child's raging disappointment at his powerless mother's response, combined with his fear of her power and rejection, contributes to the profile of a potentially dangerous child.

Mother blaming, overtly or covertly, dominates the dialogue in today's professional and public arenas. Caplan and Hall-McCorquodale (1985a, b) reviewed major clinical journals published in 1970, 1976, and 1982; documented this pattern; and concluded that it prevailed in the literature, regardless of the type of journal or the sex of the author. Mothers were consistently blamed for a wide variety of problems (Bailey, 1994). This view of mothers persists despite many studies to the contrary. As early as 1971, Schopler and Reichler found parental estimates of their autistic child's functioning across major developmental domains to be correlated significantly with professional test results. Nevertheless, the Kanner (1955) assessment of the "refrigerator mother" as a causative factor in her child's autism and the Battelheim (1967) descriptors of mothers, along with the popularity of the term the "schizophrenogenic mother" prevailed (Vosler-Hunter, 1989).

Many of these scapegoating attitudes that were evident in earlier years toward the unfortunate mothers of schizophrenic and autistic children have been transferred in the last decade to a growing group of indigent mothers of children with behavior problems. This group of very young parents, often overwhelmed and powerless in the face of day-to-day demands, has now become the official national scapegoat. Does the public need to hold onto this anger in order to justify its indifference to the plight of these children and their parents?

FEELINGS OF POWERLESSNESS ARE PERVASIVE

Frequent exposure to dangerous activities in one's community (drugs, assault, etc.) over which adults have no control also serves to increase the family's perception that they can control nothing. Combine these experiences with the inability to manage a child's unacceptable behavior, and the sense of helplessness is intensified. Since behavior management dilemmas with children have a way of making parents and even teachers feel less adequate or confident, problematic behaviors often provoke angry and punitive reactions. Dysfunctional interactions may then become the rule as overwhelmed parents struggle to deal with chronic tensions and their behaviorally disordered child. Parental reactions of impotence and anger may be exacerbated by public shaming and criticism, which minimizes their need for services.

Kagan's studies (1970) of families throughout the world reported that one of the earliest discriminators of social class is the perceived sense of control over the events in one's own life. A mentally healthy person is able to perceive of him- or herself as minimally powerful—capable of influencing the immediate environment, i.e., the behavior of one's own child in beneficial ways (Hollingshead and Redlich, 1958). Increasing control over one's destiny is an important mechanism for increasing a person's sense of competence and power (Zigler and Berman, 1983). It follows from this that empowerment contains an important psychological attribute of perceived personal confidence and control of the self, and is both an internal and external process. The internal component—the psychological attitude that one is competent to make decisions or solve one's problem—needs to be coupled with an external component, which is the actual experience of the exercise of power.

Many parents of these troubled preschoolers with disorganized families have described a sense of powerlessness that began in their own early childhood. By the time they are teenagers, these feelings are entrenched. Clearly, young children born into dysfunctional families with besieged parents struggling to deal with life-threatening circumstances do not have the same experiences as more privileged children. Babies from this background learn very early that their calls and cries are not likely to elicit a nurturing response. This sense that one has power, that one's needs and desires will be heard and will make a difference, is established or eroded very early. Children who grow up in families without the means to be responsive learn very soon that their needs and dreams do not make much of a difference. Many of these poor children give up very early. Dr. T. Berry Brazelton at a public lecture in 1991 reported reactions of hopelessness he observed in infants as young as nine months, conditioned by circumstance to understand that if they cried or fussed, it made no difference. There was nobody who was going to come to them or do something for them. As a result, patterns of powerlessness set in very early. These children grow up to become the teenage parents of the next generation. Compare this pattern to the experience of more privileged children, who learn that not only what they want for Christmas but also what they want for dinner, or what they want to do after school has a real impact.

IS THERE A PROFESSIONAL RESPONSE?

Reports that parents in communities of urban poverty are underinvolved participants in their children's preschool education (Turnbull and Turnbull, 1990) seem to place primary responsibility for participation on the parents. The process of "blaming the victim" is a familiar one. What responsibility should be assigned to the systems and the professionals that create barriers in the form of program constraints, expectations, or attitudes that interfere with involvement in the child's education? Professional assumptions, intended or unintended, about etiology and the nature of parent and child interactions may have created barriers that interfere with essential collaboration (Vosler-Hunter, 1989).

PROMISING INTERVENTIONS REQUIRE ENHANCEMENT OF THE EMPOWERMENT PROCESS

A promising approach to this problem can be found in two federally funded programs: preschool special education and Head Start. In these systems, intervention with the child and collaboration with the parents begin before it is too late and patterns are set that later may be too difficult to change.

Both Head Start and IDEA (Individuals with Disabilities Education Act, earlier known as PL 94-142 and PL 99-457) created opportunities for young children with, or at risk of, later disabilities as well as for their families. While each system targeted a different population, both considered the preschool years "critical" and proposed interventions that could promote the child's development and change feared-for outcomes. Most significantly, each program relied upon an early educational experience in combination with parental involvement to effect this change (Zigler, 1992).

Federal and state legislation and support prompted the emergence of a collection of autonomous local Head Start programs offering services as early as 1965. Decades later, Edward Zigler (1990), the "father" of Head Start, concludes that "in regard to economically disadvantaged children, a consensus now exists among behavioral scientists, policymakers and even taxpayers that early intervention is a cost-effective method for combating the effects of poverty experienced early in life." Edward Zigler and Head Start initiated a trend toward parent involvement in the child's early educational start that built upon the strengths of families. Studies of Head Start demonstrated that the children made social as well as cognitive gains, and the program also increased the family's ability to provide a more favorable developmental environment for their children.

A CLINICAL EXAMPLE:
THE HOME/SCHOOL COLLABORATIVE MODEL

A similar outcome has been documented in the effectiveness of preschool special education, in which home/school collaboration has been the cornerstone of practice. Studies provide evidence that shared power and a family-friendly system are strategies that can promote successful collaborations with parents of preschoolers with social/emotional disorders (Bloch, Hicks, and Friedman, 1994; Bloch and Seitz, 1989). An empowerment perspective with supportive linkages between home and school characterizes the Variety Pre Schooler's Workshop (VPSW) process. This model puts into practice Bronfenbrenner's (1979) proposals that child development is advanced by frequent interactions with professional providers, goal consensus between settings, and supportive linkages.

A systematic method to involve parents is initiated from the outset. It starts at the first contact for screening and evaluation to determine eligibility and placement (Bloch, 1988), moves on to the Individualized Education Program (IEP) and remediation, and ends with preparation for transition into another setting. Parents are considered indispensable members of their child's interdisciplinary team. Although the involvement is different for each family, for almost all, collaboration has been found feasible.

The Home/School Collaborative Model (HSCM) is based on three important constructs (Bloch, 1991; Spiegle-Mariska and Harper-Whalen, 1991):

- A family-friendly school system;
- Family support services and mutual aid; and
- Parental participation in assessments, goal setting, and remediation.

THE FAMILY-FRIENDLY, OPEN SCHOOL SYSTEM

The "family-friendly" school system is an "open school" (Spiegle-Mariska and Harper-Whalen, 1991). At a family-friendly school, parents are always welcome and no appointment or permission to visit is needed. One-way viewing mirrors and intercoms facilitate the observation of children in the classroom and at all therapies. Staff at the school are approachable and available for both informal and formal meetings. A parent lounge, which houses a specialized parent/professional library, provides a place for parents to network and to find respite, information, and comfort. It creates a gathering place where families can meet one another, make new friends, or simply relax. After-school and Sunday programs offer year-round respite to parents and mainstreamed social/recreational/educational opportunities for children and their siblings (Bloch and Seitz, 1985).

Family Support Services and Mutual Aid

Parents attend a series of evening orientation meetings when their child begins school (Powell, 1989). In this way, families are familiarized with the school system—the way it works and the concept and value of a home/school partnership. These sessions focus on beginnings for both the parent and the child in the preschool special education system. The child's initial task is to separate from home and adjust to school; the parents' task is to acquire more information about the team concept at the school and the collaborative model. Parents are also trained at this time in the use of The Five Ps (Parent/Professional Preschool Performance Profile) System,* a shared assessment instrument and process. These meetings alert parents to potential troublesome family issues that may emerge as a result of the presence of a child with a disability. Social workers provide a menu of family support services from which a family may choose individual, couple, or family counseling; parent education and behavior management groups; a variety of mutual-aid groups for mothers, couples, siblings, and grandparents; and after-school and Sunday recreation and respite activities.

Parent Participation in Assessment, Goal Setting, and Remediation

Shared assessment is a key aspect of the collaborative model. It begins with the appointment for a screening for a child with a suspected disability. Parents are involved in data collection and rating judgments of behaviors. The Five Ps Parent Data Questionnaire (PDQ) (Bloch, 1992) is a tool used with parents at this stage. The inclusion of parent ratings increases the accuracy of the entry-level professional multidisciplinary evaluation of a child's current level of functioning and the beginning goals (Bailey, 1989; Spiegle-Mariska and Harper-Whalen, 1991).

The Five Ps PDQ (derived from the more comprehensive Five Ps) consists of ratings of approximately 125 observed behavioral items. Parental ratings are based on their observations of their child in the home environment. Learning to use the PDQ and later the more comprehensive Five Ps Education Assessment is a tool in parent education because it helps them in the following:

---

*The Five Ps (Parent/Professional Preschool Performance Profile), published by Variety Pre-Schooler's Workshop, is an assessment instrument for children 6 to 60 months old with learning, language, or behavior problems.

- Learn to observe their child's behavior
- Systematically collect data about their child's behavior at home
- Increase their understanding of early childhood development
- Recognize behaviors that interfere with learning
- Acquire rating skills
- Develop more realistic expectations for their child
- Monitor change over time

When a child enters the school program, parents become involved in the next phase of collaboration: preparation of the more comprehensive Five Ps Education Assessment (Bloch, 1987). Parental responses to the opportunity to participate in their child's evaluation have indicated that this system has increased their understanding of their child's development and their child's disability and helped them communicate more effectively with their child's teacher (Bloch, Hicks, and Friedman, 1994). This, in turn, has facilitated collaboration and increased consensus over remediations that help the child develop the necessary inner controls. Since the most effective interventions with preschoolers take place at the site and time the incident is happening and with the key people involved (which means at home and in school), consensus between the two systems is a powerful construct in promoting the child's development.

Collaboration and Empowerment

The VPSW approach is named the Home/School Collaborative Model, but it might more accurately be termed the Home/School Collaborative and Empowerment Model. The two processes, collaboration and empowerment, are distinct, but they are very much linked. The three important components—a family-friendly, open system; family support and mutual-aid services; and parent participation in assessment, goal selection, and remediation—serve to foster both processes.

The basic rationale for promoting collaboration is based on the observation that this powerful process will enhance the parents' natural desire to help their own child and promote plans that are flexible and suited to the unique needs of each family and child (Dunst, Trivette, and LaPointe, 1994; Spiegle-Mariska and Harper-Whalen, 1991; Vosler-Hunter, 1989). The model recognizes that both parents and professionals possess critical information about the nature of the child's needs and development. Parents and professionals share a mutual goal—helping the child adapt and grow. Key elements in the collaborative process are the following:

- Mutual respect for skills and knowledge.
- Two-way sharing of information.
- Shared planning and decision making.

CONCLUDING REMARKS

"Crime," many Americans say, "is one of our country's greatest problems" (*Parade Magazine*, 1994). Violent crimes involve a disproportionate number of adolescents (Garrett, 1995). Many of these problem youngsters had disorders that were identified when they were preschoolers. Unchecked, such youngsters are more likely to become school dropouts and *eight* times more likely to become involved in delinquency. The prisons are filled with young men with reading disabilities. More than 70 percent are functionally illiterate. In 1990, nearly one-third of those arrested were people under twenty-one years of age and 1.7 million were under age nineteen. The highest ratios of violence are reported in adolescents between the ages of fifteen to nineteen (Tatge, 1995).

George Will (1987), the columnist, refers to a survey taken in the 1940s, which listed

> the top seven discipline problems in public schools. They were talking, chewing gum, making noise, running in the halls, getting out of turn in line, wearing improper clothes, not putting paper in wastebaskets. By contrast, a survey from the 1980s lists these school problems: drug abuse, alcohol abuse, pregnancy, suicide, rape, robbery, assault.

A more recent survey mentions arson, gang warfare, venereal disease, and AIDS. In other words, our schools and neighborhoods are no longer safe.

Despite this growing social crisis and the demonstrated effectiveness of early starts versus neglect and later consequences, two federally legislated and funded programs are devalued and under siege: Head Start and preschool special education. Head Start remains underfunded; only one-third of eligible children are enrolled (Carnegie Corporation, 1994). Often these children are enrolled only for one year at age four instead of for two years starting at age three, a much more effective intervention. In addition, the quality of Head Start care is jeopardized by inadequate salaries, which in turn lead to a high rate of staff turnover, an anathema to relationships with young children and parents. Despite these handicaps, the program's aim of changing the results of poverty and promoting alternative ways of solving problems for the children and families has been effective.

Preschool special education, which became a mandated entitlement in 1986 (although there were many earlier pioneers) is also under siege. Some critics contend it is too costly (although one year of incarceration costs at least as much). Others now proclaim that inclusion or mainstreaming is a Civil Rights issue and the only viable early intervention model. While there is some evidence that higher-performing students with disabilities benefit from integrated classes, lower-performing children gained more from segregated classes (Cole, 1991). The rationale and benefits of integration of preschoolers with disabilities are linked to many variables: teacher preparation, strategies and support services, environmental arrangements, and activities aimed at peers with disabilities (Demchak and Drinkwater, 1992; Wolery and Wilbers, 1994).

Anecdotal reports from schools and teachers convey serious concerns, including behaviorally disabled preschoolers who bite, hit, and hurt others. The issue in these instances is less the degree of disability and more the problem of classroom manageability. The controversy regarding placement in preschool special education continues to rage. It has been addressed by the Council for Exceptional Children (CEC) and other professional and parent groups. All conclude, however, that the preschool special education system has made contributions with far-reaching national impact, improving the educational outcome of young children with disabilities who had earlier been deprived of the benefit of schooling.

Assaults on both the Head Start and preschool special education systems seem to be motivated by short-term political considerations with unrealistic expectations. Promoting behavioral change requires a complex and sustained approach carried out consistently over a number of years. Programs with the greatest likelihood of decreasing the antisocial behavior of children will have to provide a full range of interventions, quality preschool, and support services to families.

Power and its impact were considered in both the Head Start and preschool special education legislation. Program implementation has, however, been variable. Receptivity on the part of parents and professionals to potential partnerships required trust and changed attitudes (Vosler-Hunter, 1989). Sometimes, young parents had to deal with and overcome their own earlier experiences of painful school failure before they could become collaborators. Professionals had to increase their sensitivity to attitudes that could alienate parents. The balance of power between the home/parent and school/teacher can be addressed with the Home School Collaborative Model (HSCM) and The Five Ps System. An accent on meaningful communication through the assessment and placement process promotes parental involvement and prevents disillusionment with the collaborative process (Harry, Allan, and McLaughlin, 1995).

While further controlled studies are needed to document the effectiveness of these early starts in reducing the later incidence and costs of delinquency and crime, there is already a growing body of evidence from programs across the country cited by Edward Zigler in "Early Intervention to Prevent Juvenile Delinquency," *The Harvard Mental Health Newsletter*, September 1994 that provides good preliminary evidence and points in that direction.

The experience at some Head Start centers and special education preschool programs provides evidence that shared power and a family-friendly system have benefitted many preschoolers with or at risk of social incompetence and also aided their parents. Despite the evidence that these models can play an important role in identifying and averting later problems, both systems are under siege. Support for these federally mandated programs could decrease the growing numbers of violent adolescents and reduce our prison population. The savings from the administration of an expensive criminal justice and prison system could be more wisely and effectively applied to the preschool special education system and an expansion of the Head Start program.

REFERENCES

America's biggest worries. (1994). *Parade Magazine*, (October 23), p. 6.

Bailey, D. B., Jr. (1989). Assessment and its importance in early intervention. In D. B. Bailey, Jr. and M. Wolery (Eds.), *Assessing infants and preschoolers with handicaps* (pp. 1-21). Columbus, OH: Merrill Publishing Co.

Bailey, D. B., Jr. (1994). Working with families of children with special needs. In M. Wolery and J. S. Wilbers (Eds.), *Including children with special needs in early childhood programs* (pp. 23-44). Washington, DC: National Association for the Education of Young Children (NAEYC).

Battelheim, B. (1967). *The empty fortress*. New York: The Free Press.

Bloch, J. (1971). Nonverbal messages: A means to verbalization. *Teaching Exceptional Children*, *4*(1), 10-17.

Bloch, J. (1988). Shared assessment: Another approach to the parental link. *DEC Communicator*, *15*(2) (November-December).

Bloch, J. S. (1987). *The Five P's (Parent/Professional Preschool Performance Profile*. Syosset, NY: Variety Pre-Schooler's Workshop.

Bloch, J. S. (1991). *The VPSW Home/School Collaborative Model*. Syosset, NY: Variety Pre-Schooler's Workshop.

Bloch, J. S. (1992). *The Five P's Parent Data Questionnaire (PDQ)*. Syosset, NY: Variety Pre-Schooler's Workshop.

Bloch, J. S., and Seitz, M. (1985). *Empowering parents of disabled children: A family exchange center*. Syosset, NY: Variety Pre-Schooler's Workshop.

Bloch, J. S., and Seitz, M. (1989). Parents as assessors of children: A collaborative approach to helping. *Social Work in Education*, *11*(4), 226-244.

Bloch, J. S., Hicks, J. S., and Friedman, J. L. (1994). *Home/school collaboration and parental involvement*. Syosset, NY: Variety Pre-Schooler's Workshop.

Brazelton, T. B. (November, 1991). "Touchpoints for anticipatory guidance." Presented at Variety Pre-Schooler's Workshop 25th Anniversary Confrence, Syosset, NY.

Bronfenbrenner, U. (1979). *The ecology of human development: Experiments by nature and design*. Cambridge, MA: Harvard University Press.

Caplan, P. J., and Hall-McCorquodale. (1985a). Mother-blaming in major clinical journals. *American Journal of Orthopsychiatry*, *55*(3), 345-353.

Caplan, P. J., and Hall-McCorquodale. (1985b). The scapegoating of mothers: A call for change. *American Journal of Orthopsychiatry*, *55*(4), 610-613.

Carnegie Corporation of New York. (1994). *Starting points: Meeting the needs of our youngest children*. New York: Author.

Children's Defense Fund. (1994). *The state of America's children yearbook 1994*. Washington, DC: Author.

Cole, K. (1991). Effects of preschool integration for children with disabilities. *Exceptional Children*, *58*(1), 36-45.

Demchak, M., and Drinkwater, S. (1992). Preschoolers with severe disabilities: The case against segregation. *Topics in Early Childhood Special Education*, *11*(4), 70-83.

Dunst, C. J., Trivette, C. M., and LaPointe, N. (1994). Meaning and key characteristics of empowerment. In C. J. Dunst, C. M. Trivette, and A. G. Deal (Eds.), *Supporting and strengthening families: Vol. 1. Methods, Strategies and Practices* (pp. 12-28). Cambridge, MA: Brookline Books.

Eron, L. D. (1994). It's not easy, but inner city youth can unlearn aggressive behavior. *The Brown University Child and Adolescent Behavior Letter*, (November), pp. 1-3.

Garrett, L. (1995). Murders by teens soaring. *Newsday*, (February 18), p. A11.

Harry, B., Allen, N., and McLaughlin, M. (1995). Communication versus compliance: African-American parents' involvement in special education. *Exceptional Children, 61*(4), 364-377.

Hollingshead, A., and Redlich, F. (1958). *Social class and mental illness*. New York: John Wiley.

Kagan, J. (1970). On class differences and early development. In V. Denenberg (Ed.), *Education of the infant and young child* (pp. 5-24). New York: Academic Press.

Kanner, L., and Eisenberg, L. (1955). Notes on the follow-up studies of autistic children. In P. H. Hoch and J. Zubin (Eds.), *Psychopathology of childhood*. New York: Grune and Stratton.

NAEYC Position Statement on Violence in the Lives of Children. (1993). *Young Children, 48*(6), 80-84.

Powell, D. R. (1989). *Families and early childhood programs*. Washington, DC: NAEYC.

Public Agenda. (1995). Kids who commit crimes: What should be done about juvenile violence? *National Issues Forums*. New York: McGraw-Hill, Inc.

Schopler, E., and Reichler, R. J. (1971). Parents as cotherapists in the treatment of psychotic children. *Journal of Autism and Childhood Schizophrenia, 1*, 87-102.

Spiegle-Mariska, J., and Harper-Whalen, W. (1991). *Forging Partnerships with families. Module 3.* (Report No. EC 300 922). Missoula: Montana University, Division of Educational Research and Services. (ERIC Document Reproduction Service 342 163).

Tatge, C., Executive Producer. (January, 1995). *What can we do about violence with Bill Moyers*, Parts 1 and 2. New York: Public Affairs Television, Inc.

Turnbull, A. P., and Turnbull, H. R. (1990). *Families, professionals and exceptionality,* second edition. Columbus, OH: Merrill.

Umansky, W. (1983). Assessment of social and emotional development. In K. D. Paget and B. A. Bracken (Eds.), *The psychoeducational assessment of preschool children* (pp. 417-441). New York: Grune and Stratton, Inc.

Vosler-Hunter, R. (1989). *Families as allies project* (pp. 18-24). Portland, OR: Portland State University Institute Report.

Wallach, L. B. (1994). Violence and young children's development. *ERIC Digest*, (June 1994), EDO-OS-94-7.

Will, George F. (1987). Three balls, two strikes. *Newsweek*, (January 5), p. 64.

Wolery, M., and Wilbers, J. S. (1994). Introduction to the inclusion of young children and special needs in early childhood programs. In M. Wolery and

J. S. Wilbers (Eds.), *Including children with special needs in early childhood programs* (pp. 1-22). Washington, DC: NAEYC.

Zigler, E. (1990). Foreword. In S. J. Meisels and J. P. Shonkoff (Eds.), *Handbook of early childhood intervention* (pp. ix-xiv). New York: Cambridge University Press.

Zigler, E. (1992). Early interventions to minimize delinquency. *Clinician's Research Digest: Briefings in Behavioral Science, 10*(2).

Zigler, E. (1994, September). Early intervention to prevent juvenile delinquency. *The Harvard Mental Health Newsletter*, 5-7.

Zigler, E., and Berman, W. (1983). Discerning the future of early childhood intervention. *American Psychologist*, 894-906.

Chapter 12

Cultural Diversity Among Hispanic Families: Implications for Practitioners

Carlos Vidal

HISPANICS AND THE SOCIAL WORK PROFESSION

At the time of the 1990 Census, there were approximately 25 million Hispanics in the United States, representing nearly 10 percent of the population of the nation (U.S. Bureau of the Census, 1990). Furthermore, the Hispanic population in the United States is the most rapidly expanding cultural group in the country. Whereas the population of the nation as a whole increased by less than 10 percent in the decade preceding the 1990 Census, the Hispanic population increased almost sevenfold. The large number of undocumented aliens in the nation suggests that these census figures may in fact underestimate both the number of Hispanics and the rate of increase in the proportion of the population who are Hispanic.

It should be noted that the term *Hispanic* is generally used to refer to individuals of Mexican, Central or South American, Puerto Rican, Cuban, or Dominican descent. Arbona and Novy (1991) have noted that this is an extremely diverse group:

> Hispanics differ not only in their descent but also in socioeconomic background, educational attainment, immigration status, and race. Although information on the Hispanic population as a whole provides a useful overview of this ethnic group, it also serves to mask the different experiences and problems faced by the individual subgroups. (p. 335)

Generalizations regarding Hispanic clients can be both helpful and potentially dangerous. For example, it is true that Hispanics as a group tend to be characterized by relatively low incomes. This is important because low socioeconomic status has been shown to be related negatively to individual self-concept and subjective well-doing (Coke and Twaite, 1995; Diener et al., 1985; Sherif, 1982).

The recognition of the socioeconomic disadvantages typically faced by Hispanic clients led Slavin and colleagues (1991) to recommend the following to clinicians working with Hispanic clients: "It is important to assess the individual's resources and to help them to expand and/or use available resources. This requires the counselor to look beyond the individual to the family, extended family, and community" (1991, p. 162). On the other hand, reliance on such data can result in overgeneralization and stereotyping of Hispanic clients among workers who are not familiar with specific Hispanic cultural groups. For example, Arbona and Novy (1991) pointed out that "Cubans and people from Central and South America compose a greater proportion of professional workers and attain higher levels of education than do Mexicans or Puerto Ricans" (p. 335). Thus, a fundamental guideline for those working with Hispanic clients is that it is important to recognize both the general characteristics of Hispanics as a group and the tremendous variability among the diverse cultural groups subsumed under this broad category.

Furthermore, even within specific Hispanic cultural groups, there is tremendous variability among individuals. As with clients from any cultural group, such differences reflect differences in physical characteristics, as well as environmental advantages and disadvantages. In the case of Hispanic clients, however, variability among individuals is also influenced by the process of acculturation. Marin et al. (1987) have defined acculturation with respect to Hispanics as follows:

> As a minority group, Hispanics are exposed to the mainstream cultural patterns of the United States and modifications in their values, norms, attitudes and behaviors may be expected to occur because of this contact. This process of changes in behavior and values by individuals has been labeled "acculturation" (Gordon, 1964) and refers to the culture learning that

occurs when immigrants come in contact with a new group, nation, or culture (Berry, 1980; Dohrenwend and Smith, 1962). (Marin et al., 1987, p. 184)

Acculturation has been shown to be related significantly to one's mental health status (Golding et al., 1985; Griffith, 1983; Hatcher and Hatcher, 1975).

The process of acculturation implies that even within a single specific Hispanic cultural group, one client may differ from another in a number of ways that might affect the provision of social work services. According to Casas and Vasquez (1996), the process of acculturation operates with respect to language preference and use, socioeconomic status, and culture-specific attitudes and values.

> Although the less acculturated Hispanic may speak both Spanish and English, gain lower socioeconomic status, and adhere to attitudes and values that include a strong family orientation, personalism, idealism, and informality (characterized as a more passive and humanistic orientation toward life), the more acculturated Hispanic may no longer speak Spanish, may attain middle- or upper-class status, and may strongly adhere to majority-culture values, including individualism, efficiency, and a strong orientation toward achievement (characterized as the Protestant work ethic). (p. 163)

Thus, Hispanic clients tend to differ from clients in the majority culture along several important demographic and cultural dimensions, although the extent of these differences varies greatly both across and within Hispanic subgroups. But do these differences matter in terms of the delivery of social work services? This is a subject that has generated some controversy in the field. This subject is considered in the section that follows.

THE ETIC AND EMIC PERSPECTIVES

Some experts on counseling in general (Frank, 1963) and counseling Hispanics in particular (Ibrahim, 1985) have argued that the most important principles of counseling are universal in nature, reflecting aspects of human experience that are common to all people, independent of one's culture. This viewpoint, known as the etic perspective, leads to a deemphasis of the importance of cultural differences and "the belief that counseling theories and methods can be effective regardless of culture" (Patterson and Welfel, 1994, p. 168).

In contrast, other experts have argued that counseling must be culture-specific. For example, Diaz-Guerrero (1975) called for the development of a "Mexican-American psychology." Kunkel (1990) noted that several experts had prepared detailed guidelines for counseling Mexican Americans. Kunkel suggested that these guidelines

> have been prepared under the assumption that counseling efforts with these populations must be specifically culturally sensitive and relevant (cf. Ayres, 1979; Garcia and Ybarra-Garcia, 1985, 1988; Gonzalez, 1972; Ponterotto, 1987; Szapocznik, 1986). Common to these discussions is the assumption that counseling with Mexican Americans requires a particular set of values, attitudes, and behaviors on the part of the counselor. (Kunkel, 1990, p. 286)

This view that working effectively with members of a specific cultural group requires the worker to have the values, attitudes, and behaviors of that group is known as the emic perspective. Kunkel (1990) pointed out that extreme advocates of the emic perspective even argue that an individual who is not a member of a particular cultural group cannot even conduct meaningful research on that group (e.g., Olivas, 1989).

Which of these perceptions is correct? As stated in the foregoing paragraphs, each position is probably extreme. The truth probably lies somewhere in between. However, the flaws of the extreme form of the etic perspective are perhaps more glaring than those of the emic perspective. For example, Sue and Sue (1990) pointed out that clients from minority cultural groups are less likely than clients from the majority culture to seek counseling services. Moreover, when minority clients do come to counseling, they tend to leave sooner and report less favorable outcomes. If the etic perspective were accurate, one would be hard-pressed to explain these findings.

In addition, several empirical investigations have indicated that mental health workers from the majority culture demonstrate ethnic and linguistic bias when they assign clinical diagnoses to Hispanic clients (Del Castillo, 1970; Malgady, Rogler, and Constantino, 1987; Oakland, 1977; Price and Cueller, 1981; Rosado, 1980). If cultural differences between minority-group clients and predominantly majority-group mental health workers are sufficiently large as to lead to biased diagnoses, it seems likely that these same cultural differences must have an impact on service delivery as well.

On the other hand, it seems extreme to believe that no member of a minority cultural group can ever be assisted by any worker who is not a member of that same group. Taken to the extreme, such a view could lead to the conclusion that a potential client who was a second-generation Cuban-American male whose grandparents immigrated from Camaguey and whose parents are college graduates can only be helped by a social worker with an identical demographic profile. If this is the case, it would be nearly impossible to find an appropriate professional for every individual in need of services. It is probably more appropriate to conclude, as did Ivey and Authier (1978), that the essential conditions of an effective helping relationship may indeed be universal, but the methods that majority counselors have typically been trained to use in order to establish these conditions may be wholly inappropriate for use with minority clients. Patterson and Welfel (1994) explained this as follows:

> For a client accustomed to authorities who direct and structure interaction, for example, a narrow response repertoire that is limited to clarifying, reflecting, and summarizing client comments may be so uncomfortable to the client that he or she will not be able to tolerate the ambiguity. In such circumstances, the client may misinterpret the counselor's efforts to build a trusting relationship as lack of skill or knowledge. The flexibility to take into account the client's deep assumptions about the role of an expert counselor and the usual pattern of interpersonal relationships in the client's culture is critical to the success of the counseling enterprise. (p. 176)

But what are the culturally related factors that counselors must consider when working with clients from minority cultural groups? And what are the specific cultural characteristics of Hispanic clients that must be recognized? The next section of this chapter considers these factors and characteristics.

CULTURAL FACTORS THAT INFLUENCE
THE PROVISION OF SERVICES TO HISPANIC CLIENTS

Patterson and Welfel (1994) have identified seven different aspects of human experience that are influenced by one's culture, as follows: (1) the values one holds; (2) the language one uses, including the subtle nuances of meaning that one attaches to words and idioms; (3) the intended meanings and interpretations attached to various nonverbal behavior; (4) definitions of behavior considered normal or disturbed; (5) attitudes regarding appropriate sources of help for perceived problems; (6) norms regarding family and interpersonal relationships; and (7) one's worldview, which Patterson and Welfel defined as one's "frame of reference for the making sense of one's experience and set of deep assumptions about one's relationship with the outside world" (1994, p. 168).

Scholars have explained how these factors can influence the relationship between service providers and clients from minority cultural groups. Regarding values, Nobles (1976) pointed out that white or Eurocentric culture is oriented toward individualistic goals and individual mastery, whereas other cultures emphasize the well-being of family or tribe. This cultural bias is reflected in theories of counseling that have developed in Western societies. Counselor trainees are taught to help clients achieve self-actualization. Counselors may assume that the goals and aspirations of the individual should and will take precedence over the goals and perceived interest of family or extended family. Individualism, however, is not a universal value. According to Casas and Vasquez:

> In traditional Hispanic culture, the family unit (including the extended family) is given great importance; consequently, in that cultural context it is "normal" to deal with the reality and necessity of valuing the welfare of the family higher than one's individual welfare. To speak of an individual's health and welfare independent of the health and welfare of the family unit

simply does not make good sense within traditional Hispanic culture. (1996, p. 157)

Patterson and Welfel (1994) referred to the importance of language differences. They explained that verbal communication is the "currency" of counseling, and that language barriers can represent an "enormous roadblock to effectiveness" (p. 169). These authors stressed that verbal communication is the primary way the counselor demonstrates empathic understanding, which is considered an essential element of the helping relationship in some theoretical orientations, including client-centered counseling. This observation supports the contention of Ivey and Authier (1978) that even though the essential conditions of counseling may be universal, cultural differences can affect the extent to which these conditions can be established. Patterson and Welfel (1994) also argued that language barriers increase the risk of misdiagnosis. It is possible that language differences are partly responsible for the diagnostic bias that characterizes assessments of clients from minority cultural groups made by mental health workers from the majority culture.

Regarding nonverbal behaviors, Casas and Vasquez (1996) noted that Hispanic clients may regard the counselor as an authority figure and respond in a deferential manner, often avoiding direct eye contact. An Anglo counselor who is not aware of this cultural difference may easily misinterpret such nonverbal behavior as a sign of resistance or a desire to withdraw from the counseling interview. Another example of cultural differences concerning nonverbal behavior is that Hispanics tend to be more physical than Anglos. Vidal (1993) noted that Hispanics tend to touch people with whom they are speaking. They also tend to sit or stand closer than Anglos. Hispanics generally shake hands when they meet, and they frequently engage in an introductory hug, a kiss on the cheek, or a slap on the back. Vidal advised counselors to help Hispanic clients feel comfortable by allowing them to define body space parameters. He also advised counselor to shake hands in greeting and to try to speak a bit of Spanish, even if it's just, "¡Óla! ¿Qué tal?" These apparently little behaviors can go a long way toward helping the Hispanic client overcome any fear he or she may harbor toward the counselor/authority figure.

Malgady and his associates (1987) provided an interesting example of differences between Hispanic culture and white culture concerning the definition of "normality":

> In Puerto Rican culture, it is commonplace to practice "espiritismo," or spiritualism, independent of religious affiliation (Rogler and Hollingshead, 1985). Briefly, this is an ideology positing that we are surrounded by an invisible world of spirits (good or evil) who may penetrate this world to influence human lives (e.g., cause mental illness) . . . When certain MMPI [Minnesota Multiphasic Personality Inventory] items such as, "Evil spirits possess me at times" are viewed in the context of the spiritualistic penchants of the Hispanic culture, certainly a pathological label cannot be affixed to the respondent. (p. 230)

Thus, the belief in spirits that may have a profound influence over one's life is not viewed as deviant or dysfunctional in Puerto Rican culture. It is normative. An Anglo social worker unfamiliar with espiritismo might interpret such a view incorrectly as a sign of psychosis.

This same belief system provides an example of how cultural differences influence the ways one seeks to get help for problems. Puerto Ricans who practice espiritismo are likely to seek assistance for personal or emotional problems from persons who have gained *facultades*, or psychic faculties, over the spirits. The tendency of members of some Hispanic subgroups to rely on folk healers to deal with certain categories of problems led Vidal (1993) to recommend the inclusion of such healers into the treatment plan for Hispanic clients whenever this appears to be appropriate.

In his study of Mexican-American and Anglo students in a large Southwestern University, Kunkel (1990) reported that the Mexican Americans were only one-third as likely as the Anglos to have had some prior exposure to counseling. This pattern of low utilization of mental health services is characteristic of many Hispanic subgroups. However, Kunkel also reported that prior use of counseling among the Mexican-American student sample was related significantly to level of acculturation, with prior exposure to counseling among the most highly acculturated Mexican-American group being similar to prior exposure among the Anglo sample. This observation underscores the importance of within-group differences among Hispanic groups, as well as the need to assess the level of acculturation for individual Hispanic clients.

Vidal (1993) pointed out that use of mental health services by Hispanics is influenced by a number of culturally related beliefs and values. Specifically, Hispanic clients are likely to: (1) believe that the mental health system is culturally insensitive and directed toward serving the needs of middle-class Anglos; (2) live in rural or suburban areas and/or lack the funds necessary to get to clinics and have baby-sitters during this time; (3) feel that language barriers preclude their participation in counseling with Anglo counselors; (4) feel that participation in counseling implies mental illness, which is a stigma and causes loss of respect; and (5) prefer direct, tangible, and action-oriented approaches to problems, rather than introspective "talking" approaches.

Hispanics also tend to seek help and advice within the family or extended family before seeking outside professional help. Vidal (1993) noted that in most Hispanic cultures, "[t]he strongest and most valued institution is the family, which includes the extended network of blood relatives, compadrazzo (close friends adopted as godparents), and in-laws" (p. 12). This respect for the traditional family is called familism. Provision of emotional support and advice during periods of stress is only one function of the family, which also provides financial support and care for children, the elderly, or the infirm. Vidal stressed the importance of involving family members in the treatment plans of Hispanic clients.

Concerning how cultural differences in one's view of the world can impact the provision of social work services to Hispanic clients, Patterson and Welfel (1994) pointed out that Anglo counselors with a Eurocentric cultural background tend to place great value on having a strong internal locus of control. This refers to the belief that one has the power to determine the outcomes of one's life. Hispanics, on the other hand, tend to have a relatively external locus of control in contrast to Anglos. They are more likely to have a fatalistic attitude toward life, a belief that many of the outcomes of life depend primarily on fate, luck, or historical accident. Patterson and Welfel explained that:

> A counselor with a narrow Euro-American world view would
> have a difficult time understanding or helping clients whose
> perspective on control and responsibility was at the other end
> of the continuum. Similarly, clients with an externally focused
> world view would be likely to see such a counselor's narrow
> focus on internal factors as blaming and blind to social and
> accidental influences. (1994, p. 171)

Clearly, then, culturally related differences between counselors and
clients can have a major impact on the utilization and effectiveness
of social work services among Hispanic clients. This factor argues
strongly in favor of the need to reach out to Hispanic populations in
order to promote service utilization. In view of the importance of the
church and informal social networks within many Hispanic cultures,
it is recommended that such outreach efforts work with the cooperation of preexisting community organizations.

Vidal (1993) described a number of additional characteristics of
Hispanic cultures of which Anglo counselors should be aware:
(1) *Hispanics may feel that they are outside the mainstream of
Anglo society, and that their peripheral status is the source of many
of their problems.* This same point has been made more forcefully
by Slavin et al. (1991), who suggested that minority status and the
experience of discrimination constitute sources of life stress not
experienced by the typical Anglo client. Similarly, Reynolds and
Pope (1991) referred to the "multiple oppressions" encountered by
many Hispanics, including stresses arising from cultural differences, language barriers, low levels of education and income, and in
some cases racial discrimination. (2) *Hispanics tend to adhere to
traditionally prescribed sex roles.* These traditional views of
appropriate roles for men and women may mean that it is desirable
to use counselors who are of the same sex as the client, particularly
among less-acculturated individuals. Traditional sex role stereotyping may become a source of stress as acculturation proceeds. This is
particularly the case when acculturation proceeds at different rates
among different members of the same family. There may be differences in the rate of acculturation of husbands and wives, as well as
of parents and children. Either situation can generate conflict within
the family, and counselors need to be aware of the contribution of

acculturation stress to such conflict. (3) *Hispanics place great value on children, who sometimes remain dependent on parents for longer periods of time than is typical in Anglo families.* Also, children may be expected to "follow in the footsteps of their parents" to a greater extent than is typical in Anglo families.

Given the large number of differences between Anglo culture and many Hispanic cultures, the obvious question to be addressed is, How can social workers and the social work profession respond appropriately to the challenge of diversity? This is the issue considered in the final section of this chapter.

MEETING THE CHALLENGE OF DIVERSITY WITH HISPANIC CLIENTS

For the majority Anglo counselors, the first step in the process of becoming a service provider who can be effective with clients from Hispanic cultures is developing an awareness of one's own cultural values, beliefs, and behaviors (Patterson and Welfel, 1994; Slavin et al., 1987). We all tend unconsciously to evaluate the beliefs and actions of others by reference to our own. Implicit in such comparisons may be the unconscious assumption of the inherent superiority of one's own views. Counselors must avoid falling into the trap of "cultural encapsulation" (Wrenn, 1962) by recognizing that different cultural values are not necessarily inferior, but simply different.

Second, counselors working with Hispanic clients should learn as much as possible about the cultures of origin of their clients. Note that I refer to cultures of origin (plural) rather than culture of origin, in recognition of the great diversity that exists among different Hispanic groups. A counselor working in the New York metropolitan area would be particularly interested in the Puerto Rican, Dominican, and Cuban cultures. Counselors in California or Texas would obviously have greater interest in Mexican and Mexican-American cultures. Obviously, schools of social work should provide coursework on cultural diversity. These should include content-oriented courses stressing the fundamental aspects of different cultures, as well as clinically oriented courses that help social workers become more aware of their own cultural biases and more competent in recognizing and coping with cultural differences in the practice setting.

The best way to learn about these cultures is to participate in them. Associate with members of the cultural groups with whom you work. Spend time interacting with both professionals and non-professionals from these cultures. Attend cultural festivals. Go to parties where members of these cultural groups will be present. Discuss culturally related attitudes, beliefs, and customs. Specifically, discuss the manner in which cultural differences affect your views and their views on politics and social issues.

Learn Spanish. Go to school to study Spanish, and then use it as often and as extensively as you can. Watch Spanish language television and go to Spanish language motion pictures. Read Spanish language publications, especially local publications, which will reflect the concerns of the particular client population with whom you are working.

Learn about acculturation. Learn how the process of acculturation differs from one cultural group to another. Learn about the stresses associated with the acculturation process. How does this process affect relationships between children and their parents? What about relationships between spouses? Become familiar with measures of acculturation and measures of acculturative stress that are appropriate for clients of the specific cultural groups with whom you work.

Ask clients what they expect from you, and inform them about the types of techniques that you use most often. Communicate your willingness to be flexible. Then *be* flexible. If your orientation is psychodynamic, remember that some Hispanic clients will feel more comfortable and confident with more direct forms of intervention, including specific suggestions about appropriate behavior to handle the problematic situations that arise in their lives.

Then, once you have learned all that you can about how clients from the groups you serve tend to differ from the majority culture, always remember that individual clients within these groups differ greatly from each other. Some clients from minority cultural groups will have become largely acculturated to the majority culture. Assess this dimension and proceed accordingly.

As if there were not enough variables to keep track of during a typical counseling session with a client from your own cultural group, working with clients from minority Hispanic cultures adds a whole new dimension of complexity. The more knowledge of the relevant cultural group one has, the better able one will be to cope with this complexity. However, the process is never an easy one. The key is to communicate freely with the client to clarify the cultural differences that exist between you and to determine how these differences may affect your mutual attitudes toward and expectations regarding the counseling process.

REFERENCES

Arbona, C., and Novy, D. M. (1991). Hispanic college students: Are there within-group differences? *Journal of College Student Development, 32*, 335-341.

Ayres, M. E. (1979). Counseling Hispanic Americans. *Occupational Outlook Quarterly, 23*(2), 2-8

Berry, J. W. (1980). Acculturation as varieties of adaptation. In A. M. Padilla (Ed.), *Acculturation: Theory, models, and some new findings* (pp. 9-25). Boulder, CO: Westview Press.

Casas, J. M., and Vasquez, M. J. T. (1996). Counseling the Hispanic: A guiding framework for a diverse population. In P. B. Pederson, J. G. Draguns, W. J. Lonner, and J. E. Tremble (Eds.), *Counseling across cultures* (pp. 146-176). Thousand Oaks, CA: Sage.

Coke, M. M., and Twaite, J. A. (1995). *The black elderly: Satisfaction and quality of later life.* Binghamton, NY: The Haworth Press.

Del Castillo, J. (1970). The influence of language upon symptomatology in foreign-born patients. *American Journal of Psychiatry, 127*, 242-244.

Diaz-Guerrero, R. (1975). *Psychology of the Mexican: Culture and personality.* Austin, TX: University of Texas Press.

Diener, E., Emmons, R. A., Larsen, R. J., and Griffin, S. (1985). The Satisfaction of Life Scale: A measure of global life satisfaction. *Journal of Personality Assessment, 40*, 71-75.

Dohrenwend, B. P., and Smith, R. J. (1962). Toward a theory of acculturation. *Southwestern Journal of Anthropology, 18*, 30-39.

Frank, J. D., (1963). *Persuasion and healing.* New York: Schocken.

Garcia, F., and Ybarra-Garcia, M. (1985). *Strategies for counseling Chicanos: Effects of racial and cultural stereotypes.* Olympia: Washington Office of State Superintendent of Public Instruction, Office of Equity Education. (ERIC Document Reproduction Service No. EJ 236120).

Garcia, F., and Ybarra-Garcia, M., (1988). *Strategies for counseling Chicanos: Effects of racial and cultural stereotypes.* Olympia: Washington Office of State Superintendent of Public Instruction, Office of Equity Education. (ERIC Document Reproduction Service No. ED 300687).

Golding, J. M., Burnam, M. A., Timbers, D. M., Esobar, J. I., and Karno, M. (1985). "Acculturation and distress: Social psychological mediators." Paper presented at the convention of the American Psychological Association, Los Angeles, August.

Gonzalez, C. (1972). "Counseling the Mexican-American student: A position paper." (ERIC Document Reproduction Service No. ED 101259).

Gordon, M. M. (1964). *Assimilation in American life: The role of race, religion, and national origins.* New York: Oxford University.

Griffith, J. (1983). Relationship between acculturation and psychological impairment in adult Mexican-Americans. *Hispanic Journal of Behavioral Sciences, 5,* 431-459.

Hatcher, C., and Hatcher, D. (1975). Ethnic group suicide: An analysis of Mexican-American and Anglo suicide rates in El Paso, Texas. *Crisis Intervention, 6,* 2-9.

Ibrahim, F. A. (1985). Effective cross-cultural counseling and psychotherapy: A framework. *The Counseling Psychologist, 13,* 625-639.

Ivey, A., and Authier, J. (1978). *Microcounseling: Innovations in interviewing training.* Springfield, IL: Charles C Thomas.

Kunkel, M. A. (1990). Expectations about counseling in relation to acculturation in Mexican-American and Anglo-American student samples. *Journal of Counseling Psychology, 37*(3), 286-292.

Malgady, R. G., Rogler, L. H., and Constantino, G. (1987). Ethnocultural and linguistic bias in mental health evaluation of Hispanics. *Journal of the American Psychological Association, 42*(3), 228-234.

Marin, G., Sabogal, F., Marin, B. V., Otero-Sabogal, R., and Perez-Stable, E. (1987). Development of a short acculturation scale for Hispanics. *Hispanic Journal of Behavioral Sciences, 9*(2), 183-205.

Nobles, W. W. (1976). Black people in white insanity: An issue for black community mental health. *Journal of Afro-American Issues, 4,* 21-27.

Oakland, R. (Ed.). (1977). *Psychological and educational assessment of minority children.* New York: Bruner/Mazel.

Olivas, M. A. (1989, May). An elite priesthood of white males dominates the central areas of civil-rights scholarship. *The Chronicle of Higher Education,* B1-B2.

Patterson, L. E., and Welfel, E. R. (1994). *The counseling process,* fourth edition. Pacific Grove, CA: Brooks/Cole Publishing.

Ponterotto, J. G. (1987). Counseling Mexican-Americans: A multi-modal approach. *Journal of Counseling and Development, 65,* 308-312.

Price, C., and Cuellar, L. (1981). Effects of language and related variables on the expression of psychopathology in Mexican-Americans. *Hispanic Journal of Behavioral Sciences, 3,* 145-160.

Reynolds, A. L. and Pope, R. L. (1991). The complexities of diversity: Exploring multiple oppressions. *Journal of Counseling and Development, 70,* 174-180.

Rosado, J. W. (1980). Important psychocultural factors in the delivery of mental health services to lower-class Puerto-Rican clients: A review of recent studies. *Journal of Community Psychology, 8,* 215-226.

Sherif, C. W. (1982). Needed concepts in the study of gender identity. *Psychology of Women Quarterly, 6*, 375-398.

Slavin, L. A., Rainer, K. L., McCreary, M. L., and Gowda, K. K. (1991). Toward a multicultural model of the stress process. *Journal of Counseling and Development, 70*, 156-163.

Sue, D. W., and Sue, D. (1990). *Counseling the culturally different: Theory and practice*. New York: John Wiley.

Szapocznik, J. (1986). Bicultural effectiveness training (BET): An experimental test of an intervention modality for families experiencing intergenerational/intercultural conflict. *Hispanic Journal of Behavioral Sciences, 8*, 303-330.

U.S. Bureau of the Census. (1990). *The Hispanic population of the United States: March, 1989*. (Current Population Reports, Series P-20, No. 444). Washington, DC: U.S. Government Printing Office.

Vidal, C. (1993). "Cultural implications: Treating mentally ill chemical abusers." Keynote address, seminar on cultural implications for treating the mentally ill chemical abuser. Boston, MA: Commonwealth of Massachusetts Department of Mental Health (November 15).

Chapter 13

Power Issues in Social Work Practice

Ann Hartman

It is important that social workers explore the view that the professional is inevitably political. Politics is about power and to say that the professional is political is to say that as professionals, in relationships with clients, individuals, families, groups, or communities, there is always an involvement in the dynamics of power. Sometimes social workers are very aware of it. For example, in working with "nonvoluntary clients," if there is such a thing, it is easy to recognize that there are issues of power. Child protective services or criminal justice services also bring awareness of these power dimensions. Social workers write about it, struggle with it, and feel caught between the social control functions and the social work value of self-determination.

The strong commitment to self-determination demonstrates the extent to which social workers have been concerned about the power position imbedded in their practice throughout the profession's history. Social workers started out in the late nineteenth century with the conviction that they knew how people should live. They attempted, through the use of a variety of strategies—the use of persuasion and shame, and the withholding of resources—to get people to live the way the social workers thought they should. As social work moved away from moral uplift and began to become professionalized, the concept of self-determination was embraced.

Most social workers are convinced that in their practice, they automatically honor the client's right to self-determination. This is often an illusion since many of clients can not be self-determining. True self-determination requires access to resources, access to opportunity, and access to power. Too often in this highly individualistic society in which pulling one's self up by the bootstraps is the ideal, self-determination becomes the right to be left alone, or the right to be abandoned and neglected. A growing awareness of the limitations and often the hollowness of this professional promise of client self-determination has led social workers in the past two decades to adopt the notion of empowerment. This is a more assertive view of self-determination for clients, a view which recognizes that self-determination requires power.

Client empowerment has become a goal and a slogan for the profession. However, it is not at all certain that we have examined or faced the dilemmas that emerge when a profession adopts empowerment of clients as a major goal. There has been a reluctance by social workers to look at professional power in relation to clients and to face the fact that unless workers are ready to relinquish power in work with clients, despite our good intentions, clients will remain disempowered. To examine the power of professionals is to look at the extent to which the professional is political, and to face the challenge of relinquishing power in the service of client empowerment. First, it is important to look at the sources of power and to consider the extent to which they operate in the dynamics between workers and clients.

TYPES OF POWER

Physical strength and size is the most primitive form of power and a very important one. Physical force and power is further accentuated through the acquisition of weapons. Armed struggles are escalating significantly in American society. This kind of power has little relevance for most of social work practice.

The second is the source of power found in the control of needed, required, or necessary resources. When someone has control of something that another needs or requires, he or she has power over the person in need. In its history, social work has used the control of needed resources to manipulate clients toward behavioral change. One reason that many social workers supported the separation of services from income maintenance in the 1962 amendments to the Social Security Act of 1935 was because they felt services should be offered with no strings attached. People would then be free to refuse services if they did not want them. Of course, what was not anticipated was that with the separation, funding for services would be sharply cut. There is now a complete change of the philosophy in public social welfare policy. We are experiencing a return to the nineteenth century. The change is expressed in most of the new welfare "reform" proposals, which recommend that the giving and withholding of support be used planfully and intentionally to shape and control the behavior of public assistance clients. If public policy is enacted to result in such manipulative programs, social workers will face extreme conflict between fundamental professional values and the controlling and punitive direction taken by new social welfare policy.

The third source of power is the power of position. This represents legitimate power in which institutions and their representatives are given, through legislative enactments, certain powers in particular situations. Social workers have that kind of legitimate power when they are employed in public agencies to facilitate or enact legal or legislative mandates, for example, in child protective services.

The fourth source of power is personal influence, the power exerted by charm, attachment, or persuasion. In our professional work, the most dramatic example of that is found in the use of the transference. The development and use of transference is an enormously effective way to empower therapists, hopefully in behalf of the client and to bring about positive change. No matter how well-intended, or how helpful, transference places a great deal of power in the hands of the therapist and tends to disempower clients.

Finally, the fifth source of power is one cherished by all professions, that is expertise and knowledge, or occupying the position to define the truth. The power of expertise exists at the heart of our professional practice, but it is the power source with which social workers tend to be the least aware.

These different sources of power are not discrete. They overlap and reinforce each other. For example, men are physically bigger and stronger than women. Men, particularly white men, control most of the access to resources. They hold most of the legitimate positions of power and, until recently, have had undisputed control of the definition of knowledge and truth. They may or may not use interpersonal power. They generally do not have to, as they do not need it. It is possible that the whole issue of power is very much related to women's primary interest in relationships, as presented in the work of Carol Gilligan (1982) and others of the Stone Center (Miller, 1976). The primary source of power women have is to gain influence through relationship. Traditionally their access to power has been through their relationship with men. As interpersonal influence has been women's primary survival strategy, it is not surprising that they place high value on relationships.

Social workers have been aware of the first four sources of power but have tended to be less aware of the power of professional expertise. In order to explore this fifth source of power, there must be consideration of social constructivism and postmodernism and their challenge to the profession's use of this kind of power. First, postmodernism should be reviewed. The epistemological revolution that has been taking place in the sciences and social sciences is now beginning to be felt in social work.

POSTMODERNISM AND SOCIAL CONSTRUCTIVISM

For over a century, science and the social sciences have operated on John Locke's assumption that it is possible to know the world, that one can accurately determine the "truth," the nature of reality. The major tenet of research has been that the scientific method can lead us to determine the truth through objective study and through isolating, describing, measuring, and counting variables. In the twentieth century, the comfortable assumption that we can know the world began to be challenged in physics by the theory of relativity, which generated other related developments in physics and shook the Newtonian view of the world to its foundation. The Lockean epistemology began to be challenged in every field: in biology by Maturana and Verella (1986), in anthropology by Bateson (1972) and Gaertz (1983), in sociology by Berger and Luckmann (1966), in psychology by Bruner (1986) and Gergen (1985), to mention a few. Everywhere we look, even in the mental health professions (McNamee and Gergen, 1992) and in social work (Laird, 1993), postmodern thinking is challenging our truisms.

Although all of these writers take a somewhat different position, the fundamental conception is that we cannot know objective reality beyond our perception of it. Therefore, all knowing requires an act of interpretation, or, as Bateson said, "The map is not the territory." Human beings, individually and collectively, organize and interpret their experience so that it makes sense, so that it is coherent. They do that through languaging it, through narrativizing it, through putting together stories about the way the world works that make sense. Obviously, therefore, the observer cannot be separated from the observed. Standpoint research makes this point clear (Swigonski, 1993). Further, because human beings are deeply immersed in social, cultural, and political contexts, their truths, the interpretations which they make, and their constructions of reality emerge out of and are shaped by that context. Clearly, there are multiple truths just as there are multiple observers.

What does that have to do with social work practice? What does it have to do with power and empowerment? To answer this question, we must turn to the work of Michel Foucault (1980), who teaches that not all stories are equal. It was his view that the social processes which produce what comes to be recognized as the dominant discourse, or the dominant truths, are the constructions of those in power. In fact, it was his conviction that power and knowledge are so inseparable that he referred to them as one entity—"power/knowledge." Those in power define the truth, and in turn, the truth supports those in power. We are all in some relationships in which we have more power and thus we define the truth. We are also in relationships where we have less power; thus, our truths are defined by others.

Foucault studied the development and institutionalization of what he termed "global unitary knowledges," which, through a struggle over time, have come to subjugate entire sets of knowledges, including local, indigenous, and ancient knowledges, disqualifying them as beneath the required level of scientificity. An example of this can be found in the social work literature. Years ago, social work literature often consisted of a fairly brief discussion of an issue followed by one or two detailed case examples. Approximately two decades ago, social work became more sensitive to the demands of science with a capital "S." It was felt that such "N's of one," although close to the lived experience of clients and practitioners, were not "scientific knowledge," and case narratives all but disappeared from the professional journals.

As editor of *Social Work*, I tried to find materials that reported the lived experience of clients and workers. However, the voices and stories of individual workers had been subjugated, and social workers had stopped writing and submitting such material. In time, people became aware of the change in editorial policy and a few case narratives began to trickle in. It was difficult, however, since such materials had been defined by those in power in the profession as beneath the "required level of scientificity" and exiled from the legitimate domains of formal knowledge.

Foucault's concern was not only with the centralized political, economic, and institutional regimes that produce privileged knowledge, but also with their exercise of power in the capillaries, as they flow out and are practiced at the local level. The knowledge that circulates in this way is employed in everyday interactions of submission and domination. This can best be understood through example. Let us consider that powerful, global unitary body of knowledge, the *Diagnostic and Statistical Manual of Mental Disorders*, fourth edition (DSM-IV), which is centrally established and encoded in economic, medical, and educational institutions. It is practiced at the most local level in the relationship between the social worker and the client. When a social worker is required, either by the agency's funding needs or by the rules of third-party payers to attach a diagnostic label to a client, a powerful and privileged classification system has entered the relationship. In all likelihood, this classification has affected the worker's thinking, the worker-client relationship, and the client's self-definition.

It is also important to remember that these global unitary knowledges, like the DSM-IV, these dominant discourses, are not merely descriptive; they are also prescriptive. They not only describe behavior, but they also are crucial systems of social control, prescribing the proscribing specific kinds of behaviors.

Dominant discourses, however, are not immutable. Foucault writes about how global unitary knowledges may be challenged by such terms as "an insurrection of subjugated knowledge." For example, the lived experiences, the truths of African-American women were not available to us; they did not exist in the body of formal, recognized knowledge. Recently, however, there has been an insurrection of that knowledge, primarily through literature. We gain this knowledge not only through the current literature that brings to us the lived experience of African-American women today, but also through the resurrection of historical literature, which brings forth information about the experience of African-American women three or four generations ago. African-American Studies, Women's Studies, and other marginalized bodies of knowledge are challenging the canon of the universities, the approved knowledge of college curricula that primarily includes the work and the worldviews of white European men. These areas of subjugated knowledge are usually marginalized and underfunded on campuses. They are almost always disempowered in the academic world and are not given departmental status while the canon of white Western primarily male knowledge continues to provide the core of the university experience in the United States. Certainly it is important and valuable to be exposed to this rich body of knowledge, but it is not the only knowledge. It is not the whole truth.

To turn to examples closer to social work's professional experience, the incest story is perhaps the most dramatic. It is a fascinating story of power/knowledge. In Freud's early years of practice, almost all of the women he worked with reported that they had been sexually abused as children. Thus, in one of his early papers, he presented the theory that sexual abuse in childhood was the cause of hysteria and mental and emotional disturbance in adult women. This view was extremely controversial, and there was probably a great deal of pressure placed on Freud from those who challenged his interpretation. Before long, he retracted that theory and announced that these reports from women were not relating real experiences but memories of childhood fantasies and wishes. This view was embraced by his followers and for almost 100 years, knowledge of the real experience of childhood sexual abuse was subjugated. This dominant discourse was so powerful that women themselves denied their own experience and believed the experts who told them that they were remembering their childhood fantasies, that it did not really happen.

After almost a century, the women's movement brought forth an insurrection of subjugated knowledge. Women got together in consciousness-raising groups and began to share their experiences and began to validate each other's truths. They raised their voices, and their voices changed the thinking about incest. It is important to note that it was not scientific research, but the voices of women that brought about this major change.

Another example is to be found in the definition of homosexuality as a disease in the old DSM. This definition was challenged by the insurrection of subjugated knowledge that was a part of the gay liberation movement. Another is the widely held notion of the schizophrenogenic mother or family, which was challenged by the Alliance for the Mentally Ill and other families struggling with mental illness.

In the social work profession, one of the major examples of the power of the dominant discourse and its challenge is to be found in the theories about adoption that were widely held by "experts" in the field. The adoption story, which formed the base for adoption practice until quite recently, proposed that adoption should be made to be, as much as possible, like biological parenting. In order to do this, the birth family had to be completely cut off from the adoptee through closed adoption. Further, it was felt that if an adoptee showed any interest in his or her biological roots, it was a sign that the person was troubled and the adoption unsuccessful. The women who gave birth to and relinquished their children were thought to be able to "forget," to put the birth of the baby behind them and go on with their lives. In the adoption rights movement, adoptees, birth parents, and some adoptive parents gathered together and told their stories, stories that were vastly different from the "expert knowledge" about adoption. They reported their lived experience, they raised their voices, and they changed the face of adoption practice in this country although, thus far, they have not yet been able to change the laws in many states.

bell hooks (1989), an African-American woman who has commented widely about "voice" and about the insurrection of subjugated knowledge wrote the following:

> Moving from silence into speech is for the oppressed, the colonized, the exploited, and those who stand and struggle side by side, a gesture of defiance that heals, that makes new life, new

growth possible. It is that act of speech, of "talking back," that is no mere gesture of empty words, that is the expression of our movement from object to subject—the liberated voice. (p. 9)

Thus, there is a painful paradox in being a professional committed to empowerment. A key aspect of the definition of a profession is the possession and use of knowledge and expertise. As professionals, we are supposed to be experts, but paradoxically, the power of our expertise can silence clients' voices, can disempower them, and thus subvert the goals of our profession. Social work is, however, better off than most higher status professions in this regard. This marginalized position as a low-status profession has been an advantage as it has maintained a closeness to clients. The more social work has attempted to become a mainstream, high-status profession, the more it has looked to established institutions for recognition, the farther we get away from our clients. Bertha Reynold, an outstanding, progressive social worker and teacher, taught us that.

RECOMMENDATIONS FOR SOCIAL WORK PRACTITIONERS AND EDUCATION

What must be done? First, the role of expert should be abandoned and be replaced by what has been called by some the "not knowing" position. This means ceasing to privilege our truths and bracketing our truths and theories, so that they can be put aside. When we start with a commitment to theories and truths, we will hear only what supports them rather than what challenges them. This results in leaving our social fingerprints all over our assessments.

For example, when working with a client from a different racial or ethnic group, the social worker cannot be an expert on the client or the client's ethnic group. The client is the expert. Further, the worker cannot be an expert on the particular and idiosyncratic way in which the individual or family may have adapted, made use of, and drawn upon their culture. The way that social work schools have attempted teaching ethnic-sensitive practice has been through introducing content about different ethnic groups. I believe this is a grave error that results in the teaching of stereotypes. The understanding of culture is complex. Within a group, differences are as great as between groups. There is a tendency, however, because of time constraints, to teach that large ethnic and racial populations are undifferentiated. We may teach about "the" Asian-American family without regard for the great diversity within that group consisting of many cultures, languages, religions, and histories.

Students should be taught to be informed rather than "knowing listeners." They should be taught how to listen for cultural data and how to hear it. We should teach social workers to be anthropologists, ready for a field trip, knowing where culture is to be found, in narratives, in stories, in rituals, and in values.

Second, there must be recognition that theories and the practice context are not exempt from the dominant culture in which we live, and from the dominant discourse. One dramatic example of this comes out of my experience as a young worker. I was working in a family counseling agency with a depressed housewife and mother of three children. I learned from the female psychoanalyst that this client was disturbed because she had not relinquished her phallic strivings. She was not a mature feminine woman as she had been unable to abandon her own ambitions and find full satisfaction in the achievement of her husband and children. This was 1954 and the "cult of true womanhood" was being passed on as "the truth," as "science." As a good novice, I translated this revealed wisdom into my practice.

We must deconstruct theories by looking at the context in which they developed. We must ask the questions "Who says?", "Under what circumstances?", and "Who has been advantaged by it?" The theory about women that shaped my practice with this client in 1954 was developed by a Victorian Viennese psychiatrist who admitted that women were a mystery to him. His cultural fingerprints are all over this vision of women. It is also important to consider the culture of the early 1950s. The war was over, men had returned home and "Rosie the Riveter," had to go back into the kitchen and out of GI Joe's job. The 1940s had been a period of vastly expanded options for women as they went to work and into the armed forces. This was a major social change, which occurred with great rapidity and challenged established values and power positions. The dominant discourse stated that it was essential that the nation return to traditional family life. Those controlling power/knowledge supported the return to the previous status quo and thus postponed the development of the women's movement. The psychological theories ascendent at that time supported these socioeconomic and political purposes. The seeds of women's liberation, however, were sown in the 1940s and began to bear fruit almost a generation later.

Moving to the present, one may examine the dominant discourse about recipients of Aid to Families with Dependent Children. "They're lazy. They don't want to work and they rip off the welfare system. Further, they're poor parents and are likely to be on drugs." This powerful dominant discourse, widely considered to be "the truth," is a global, unitary, totalizing characterization of a large and very varied group of people, most of them women. It is currently being used to justify the dismantling of the welfare system. It is essential to deconstruct this discourse, to expose the biases, to surface the knowledge that has been subjugated about the lived experience of many of the people on welfare that do not fit this global discourse. It is the social work profession's task to join with clients and give voice to alternate narratives based on our extensive and varied lived experiences with these women.

What does the recognition that the professional is political mean for practice? What will practice look like as we seriously adopt the goal of empowerment and if we refuse to join the forces that disempower and oppress clients? These are the forces that subjugate their knowledge and deny their realities.

First, social workers must face the fact that their practice is not exempt from the power of the ideology of the dominant discourse. We must examine the way power operates in practice and recognize with bell hooks that if we interpret the experiences, the narratives of oppressed people through our own lenses and biases, if we privilege our truths, we colonize the other (hooks, 1989). We must deconstruct our own position, our own theories, and question how we may be contributing to the oppression of our clients.

Second, practice must be a collaborative process, a process of coconstruction in which client and worker participate fully.

Third, because of this collaboration, both worker and client change in the process.

Fourth, the client must be considered the expert on him- or herself.

Fifth, there must be no place for secrets. All information and interpretations must be shared and the worker's knowledge and interpretations must not be privileged over the client's.

Finally, to paraphrase bell hooks, the work of any social worker committed to the full self-realization of clients is to take a position that is necessarily and fundamentally radical, which recognizes that practice is not neutral and that to practice in a way that liberates, that expands consciousness, that awakens, is to challenge domination at its very core.

REFERENCES

Bateson, G. (1972). *Steps to an ecology of mind*. New York: Ballantine.

Berger, P., and Luckmann, T. (1966). *The social construction of reality*. New York: Doubleday.

Bruner, J. (1986). *Actual minds: Possible worlds*. Cambridge, MA: Harvard University Press.

Foucault, M. (1980). *Power/knowledge: Selected interviews and other writings*. New York: Pantheon Press.

Gaertz, C. (1983). *Local knowledge: Further essays in interpretive anthropology*. New York: Basic Books.

Gergen, K. (1985). The social constructionist movement in modern psychology. *American Psychologist*, 40: 317-329.

Gilligan, C. (1982). *In a different voice*. Cambridge, MA: Harvard University Press.

hooks, bell. (1989). Talking Back: Thinking Feminist, Thinking Black. New York: South End Press.

Laird, J. (1993). *Revisioning social work education*. Binghamton, NY: The Haworth Press.

Maturana, H., and Varella, F. (1986). *The tree of knowledge: The biological roots of understanding*. Boston: New Science Library

McNamee, S., and Gergen, K. (1992). *Therapy as social construction*. Newbury Park, CA: Sage.

Miller, J. B. (1976). *Toward a new psychology of women*. Boston: Beacon Press.

Swingonski, M. (1993). Feminist standpoint theory and the question of social work research. *Affilia*, 8: 171-183.

White, M., and Epston, D. (1990). *Narrative means to therapeutic ends*. New York: Norton.

Index

Page numbers followed by the letter "t" indicate tables.